PET LOSS
and CHILDREN

PET LOSS
and CHILDREN

Establishing a Healthy Foundation

Cheri Barton Ross

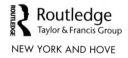

Routledge
Taylor & Francis Group

NEW YORK AND HOVE

Published in 2005 by
Routledge
270 Madison Avenue
New York, NY 10016
www.routledgementalhealth.com

Published in Great Britain by
Routledge
27 Church Road
Hove
East Sussex BN3 2FA U.K.
www.routledgementalhealth.co.uk

Library of Congress Cataloging-in-Publication Data
Ross, Cheri Barton.
    Pet loss and children : establishing a healthy foundation / Cheri Barton
Ross. — 1st ed.
        p.   cm.
    Includes bibliographical references and index.
    ISBN 0-415-94919-X (pbk. : alk. paper)
    1. Pet owners—Psychology. 2. Pet loss—Psychological aspects.
    3. Bereavement—Psychological aspects. 4. Children and animals. I. Title.

SF411.47.R6845 2005
155.9'37—dc22
                                                            2004018882

We are born helpless. As soon as we are fully conscious we discover loneliness. We need others physically, emotionally, intellectually; we need them if we are to know anything, even ourselves.

—C. S. Lewis (*The Four Loves,* 1898)

To
My Four Loves~
Mark,
Barrett, Tyler, and Savannah

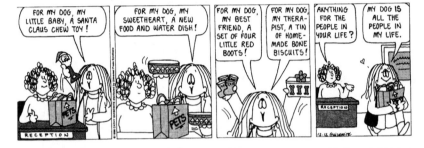

Cartoon by Cathy Guisewite reprinted with permission.

Contents

Foreword

Pet loss is often a child's first experience with death, and it provides an opportunity for adults to help children with this most intimate experience of dealing with the end of a loved one's life. Grief has many faces—anxiety, fear, sadness, guilt, regret, pain, and emptiness. Assisting children to navigate the terrain of grief will provide them with tools to cope as losses of all kinds confront them over their life span—other deaths, moves, separation or divorce, job insecurity or loss, illness or disability.

Pet Loss and Children: Establishing a Healthy Foundation is an invaluable resource for therapists, parents, and anyone who works with children when a pet dies or has to be euthanized. Therapists and professionals who work with children will want to keep this book as a handy reference when a child or family presents with pet loss as part of the therapeutic picture. Read this book from cover to cover, or choose the chapters as needed. As with any specialty, pet loss can present even the most seasoned grief counselor with challenges that require supervision or outside assistance. This book addresses in detail the many situations a counselor can encounter with pet loss so that the counselor can assist the child and family in moving through their grief. Even professionals can be tempted to trivialize pet loss, particularly if the pet was small or exotic or owned for a short period of time. It can be hard for some adults to relate to the depth of feeling a child can experience over the loss of a beloved fish, hamster, or snake. Cheri gives examples with the rule of thumb that the child's valuation of the creature is taken as paramount—as a sound bite it might be stated, "Don't flush the fish!" The death of even the smallest creature is an opportunity to assist a child with his or her feelings and questions about death according to the child's stage of development—emotional and cognitive. Details about these childhood stages of development and what the professional may see as expressed or hidden grief are given in factual information and in the many case studies Cheri presents.

Death and dying issues can be difficult for parents and caregivers of children to face, as many of us have not resolved our own issues around loss. Perhaps it is simply a deeper layer of a past loss that revisits us when a pet dies and we try to focus on helping our children. This book will help adults to identify their own feelings and loss histories, and it will guide them in identifying in a variety of loss situations what signs, symptoms, and feelings to look for in children. As we are instructed on any airplane flight, in the case of an emergency, first put on your own oxygen mask, and then assist your child.

Cheri is like a compassionate guide who sits by you in these pages, helping you to address the child's concerns as they come up. This clear communication lays a healthy foundation for moving through the feelings that loss has stirred, and for handling future losses in a successful manner. When children's feelings are validated, no matter what the feelings are, children can learn to handle their responses to any situation. With loving guidance, they will bloom into teens and adults who are not frozen in the face of life's greatest challenges.

The death of a pet provides so many opportunities for those who can make use of them. Opportunities are presented to share deep feelings and stories of the beloved pet, which helps families to bond at this difficult time. This kind of sharing about a family pet translates to handling other losses, whether past or present, regarding other family members and friends who have died. Family members can learn how to memorialize together and put their grief into positive action, not just at funeral time but also in daily life with the sharing of memories or donations to a shelter or organization. Perhaps a new life path is born of reinvesting interest in life again as a tribute to the one who is gone. After the death of a pet, children, now older, may decide to take horseback riding instruction or art lessons or to do something that has meaning to them now that their home lives and routines have had a significant change. Teaching about philosophical, spiritual, or religious beliefs, if any, can be very important when pet loss occurs. Helping children to keep the memory of the pet alive in their hearts can be modeled by adults who share their own appropriate feelings, keep pictures of the pet around, visit the grave site or have a special place for the ashes, and share memories of life with the pet. Again, we are laying the groundwork for future losses. As adults, we often know how the death of a parent, spouse, or child causes us to deal with our feelings and to keep the loved one in our heart over time. Finding one's own individual way to grieve is of paramount importance, and no one should feel ashamed of his or her own unique way of connecting to the departed.

Activities that make one feel closer to the deceased such as talking to the deceased, writing letters or poetry, or drawing are healthy ways of coping with the loss. These methods and others should be modeled by parents and shared with children, and parents should encourage children to express their opinions and feelings and to ask questions. Pet loss provides the basis on which to build for future losses, which find all of us as we age and loss becomes more prevalent.

You may find yourself recalling pet losses that were trivialized when you were a child, or perhaps as an adult. Cheri's book advocates treating each child, each feeling, and each loss situation with the greatest respect and admiration for the courage it takes to be genuine and vulnerable. Children are excellent at being genuine and vulnerable as long as they are in an environment that safely nurtures their concerns, validates their feelings, and provides a fair forum for their questions. This book was written to assist children and the child that still lives in all of us as we lose a cherished member of the family, our dear pet.

DEBORAH ANTINORI, M.A., R.D.T., L.P.C.
Author of *Journey Through Pet Loss*

Preface

As high as we have mounted in delight,
In our dejection do we sink as low.
—William Wordsworth

As deeply as children love their pets is as intensely they will experience the loss of those pets.

Explaining death to children is often an uncomfortable experience for parents and educators. Adults may feel ill at ease facing their own mortality and are generally uncertain of how to approach the topic with their children. Children can suffer in silence, and their questions about life and loss can go unanswered. Children might repress their fears, often internalizing them. They may blame themselves for the loss, or they may blame others.

Depending on their age and stage of development, children can have limited understanding of what death entails. They may not know that death is permanent—forever. Children need special support and understanding in working through a loss. Because a pet typically lives only one fifth as long as a person, it is realistic to expect that the death of a pet is one of the first losses a child will encounter. It is necessary for the healthy development of the child that a caring adult work with the child through the loss of a pet. Questions need to be answered, and children need to feel safe expressing their concerns and fears regarding death and loss. They need to be educated and supported in the pet loss experience. Laying a healthy foundation with a first loss will assist the child in becoming a mature person who has many of the tools necessary for working through other losses that will occur throughout his or her lifetime.

Death is the final stage of life. Educating a child about the death process is as important as educating a child about the birth process and human development. Death completes the cycle of life. Although beliefs regarding creation and afterlife vary among different cultures, this book respectfully addresses the topic of helping children say good-bye to their pets while encouraging parents and guardians to discuss any spiritual beliefs they may have.

Although the loss or death of a pet is not unlike other human losses, there are differences that need to be taken into consideration. The main difference is that pet loss is often an unrecognized loss in our society. It is because of this fact that addressing this type of loss is vital in providing a child with tools that will enable him or her to work through future losses. Too often, society fails to recognize the loss of a pet as being significant in a child's life. Unfortunately, children who lose pets discover that the loss is trivialized instead of being recognized as emotionally significant. The goal of any person assisting a child should be to find out what the pet means or meant to the child, and to acknowledge the relationship shared with the pet and validate the depth of the loss the child feels. Once this is understood, the caregiver can assist the child in fully working through the loss.

This book is designed to assist therapists, physicians, other health care professionals, parents, educators, and anyone who works with children in helping children through the loss of a pet. The caregiver will learn the following:

- how children grieve and how that grief is expressed in various developmental stages of understanding grief and loss,
- how to prepare children for the death of a pet,

- how to recognize hidden grief in children,
- how to address the topic of euthanasia with children,
- the importance of children's attachment to a pet and the significance of the loss,
- how to help children build a foundation from which to successfully grieve and work through loss,
- pet loss as a family experience and to share grief and feelings,
- how to help children through a sudden and unexpected pet loss,
- how to assist children through multiple losses, and
- the types of therapies and approaches used in assisting a grieving children.

I hope that those who have children or work with them will use this book as a resource. One of the greatest rewards for a caregiver is to help a child to develop to his or her fullest potential. We all hope that our children will grow into adults who have the skills, tools, and understanding necessary to maintain mental health and the ability to love and let go throughout their lives.

I know that in my own work in establishing and running a pet loss support group for the past 15 years, I have had the privilege to meet and assist caring people who have struggled with the loss of their pets. Often, adults in the group will recall the first pet loss they experienced during childhood and share feelings associated with the loss. Many times there are unresolved feelings because adults did not take their loss seriously.

The recent loss of a pet can be an opportunity to work through past losses. In working with pet owners and therapists, I have seen that the topic of children and pet loss is one that needs to be addressed in depth. Doing so will give future generations a firm foundation to build on when going through the many losses that people have to endure in a lifetime.

I have enjoyed working with the children who have attended the group I lead. Their honesty and heartfelt emotions about their pets and what the loss means to them have helped many adults in the groups as well. I offer my thanks to those parents who care so deeply about their children that they seek out support and information about loss in order to assist them. It takes courage to face a loss. Loving and letting go is a part of life. It is with great respect for the pet owners with whom I have worked over many years that I wrote this book, with the hope that other therapists can assist their clients and that parents and caregivers can effectively assist their children through a loss.

I have learned so much from the many pets with which I have been blessed to share my life, and I have been even more blessed by my three children, who love animals too.

Although this book specifically addresses pet loss, it would be foolish to not address the issues that surround loss in general. Loss occurs in many forms. One of the issues we address in this book is the loss of feeling safe. One way to help children to feel safe when their world is shaken is to show them how to reach out to others during a stressful time. When 9/11 happened, although the attacks on the United States happened on the other side of the country, far from our California home, the children at my children's elementary school—Mark West Elementary School—felt frightened and uncertain. At back-to-school night the children's artwork and papers contained variations of planes flying into buildings, smoke, flames, and people in distress. As much as we try to protect children from witnessing or hearing about such horrors, children do hear, and as a result they experience the feelings associated with such a loss. The children's school didn't dismiss or minimize their fears. The staff addressed them and helped the children by encouraging them to take positive action and to reach out to children on the East Coast who lived near the attacks. One person I want to especially thank for creating and organizing a teddy bear drive is Diane

Baird. She found a way to assist the children in working through their own anxieties by helping to make a difference in the lives of the children who were directly affected by 9/11.

In addition, I give a heartfelt thank-you to Janet Kirk, a third-grade teacher at Mark West Elementary School, for her friendship and for assisting me, along with her class, in sharing their pet loss stories and much of the artwork in this book. Also, I give a thank-you to Mark West School District superintendent Peggy Greene and principal Jennifer Bylund, who support this project. I extend my gratitude to Kathy Coker, principal at Santa Rosa Middle School, and the students who contributed stories, poetry, and artwork about pet loss.

I want to thank several other special people who helped in the completion of this book: Emily Epstein Loeb, my editor at Taylor & Francis, who believed in this project from its inception, and Brook Cosby, who expertly guided it through to publication. Marsha Calhoun's enthusiasm for this project and expertise in editing is appreciated.

Also, a thank-you goes to Jane Sorensen, my coauthor for our book *Pet Loss and Human Emotion: Guiding Clients Through Grief,* who assisted me with some the case examples and therapeutic information in this book, and, most important, is a lifelong friend. You have always taught me that when a door closes, pound on all the others until you find one that opens.

Therapist and very good friend Deborah Antinori's honesty, insight, and suggestions helped me to fine-tune the manuscript and provide a poignant title for this book. A thank-you goes to psychotherapist David Grand for assisting with the eye movement desensitization and reprocessing information. Racelle LaMar, D.V.M., deserves a heartfelt acknowledgment for continuing to keep the Redwood Empire Veterinary Medical Association (REVMA) Pet Loss Support Group funded and for her support for this project. The work of my husband, Mark A. Ross, D.V.M., has inspired me to pursue a deeper understanding of the bonds people share with their pets. His wonderful bedside manner with both his patients and clients includes referring them to the REVMA Pet Loss Support Group.

A heartfelt and warm thank-you goes to the children (including my own) who contributed to this book through their stories, artwork, and poetry. May you continue to know, throughout your lifetime, the unconditional love that animals provide.

1
PET LOSS
A Family Experience

Change is the law of life.
—John F. Kennedy

There is a time for everything, a season for every activity under
heaven. A time to reap, a time to sow, a time to gather together
and a time to let go, a time to be born and a time to die.
—Ecclesiastes 3:1

Children grow up witnessing change in nature. They learn
that there is a natural rhythm and flow to life. They watch
the leaves grow on the trees, see them go from green to red
to brown and then fall from the branches. They watch as the
barren land becomes covered with snow. They feel the tem-
perature change and then witness the process of rebirth and
death every year that they are alive. With change comes an-
ticipation, sometimes with dread and sometimes with joy for
the good things that it brings (such as butterflies or snow-
flakes). Children of any age can feel the discomfort of the
bitter cold on their bodies and the pelting rain against their
cheeks. As they grow older they often learn that even the
worst of thunderstorms brings rainbows afterward. Before
children can even articulate the changes they witness around
them, they have come to accept them as part of the cycle of

1

life. From this knowledge, children can build on a foundation of the cycle of life that includes the birth of people and animals and the death of both as well.

As children grow, they realize that there is sadness in death, in having to say good-bye. Whether it's a matter of losing the beautifully colored leaves on the trees or losing a loved one, sharing discomfort and sadness can help to cement family ties and bring children, their parents, siblings, and extended family closer together. This is one of the positive changes that can occur through experiencing loss. Any change, even if for the better, is accompanied by discomforts, and learning to comfort each other through the loss of a beloved pet can assist children by helping them to feel important, cherished, and cared for within a family structure.

The child's relationship with a pet determines the level of grief he or she will feel with the loss of that pet. Understanding the relationship children share with pets is the first step in helping them to work through a loss. To assist children through the loss of a pet, we must first take the time to understand what pets may mean to children.

A child of any age can bond with and develop an attachment to an animal. Terry Levy, Ph.D., and Michael Orlans, M.A., in their book *Attachment, Trauma and Healing,* described bonding as a physical and psychological connection that can last a lifetime.[1] They explained that attachment is the enduring emotional connection characterized by the development of trust, security, and the desire for closeness, particularly when the child is under stress. Although they described the relationship between parent and child, the same principles of attachment and bonding can be related to child and pet.

Attachment Theory

Emotionally healthy children are able to demonstrate affection toward those they care about. They seek comfort from

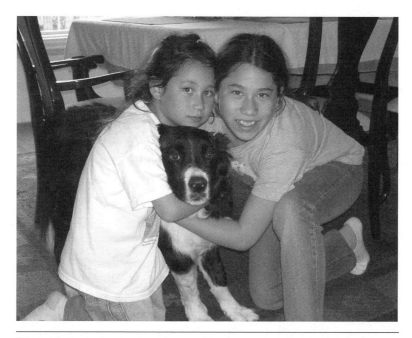

Figure 1.1 Stephanie and Jessamine love Shlomo like a member of their family.

those they trust when they are feeling bad. They are able to help themselves appropriately for their cognitive age and are willing to ask for help when they need it. They are cooperative with caregivers without being excessively demanding or demonstrating an excessive lack of cooperation. They often check in with those in charge when exploring unfamiliar territory (either through play or in a new environment). Children who love their animals will be affectionate with them. They might comfort the pet when it is hurt or frightened. They might provide food, shelter, and water for their pets (appropriate for the children's abilities). Although the majority of children have a healthy attachment to their pets, it is important to note that children who turn to their pets consistently for affection and comfort are children who are not able to get their needs met in their home environment. Therapists who work with children whose pets are at the center of their lives need to fully explore the family dynamics.

Relationships Children Share with Their Pets

A pet can be a wonderful friend to a child. Often cute, cuddly, playful, and loving, a pet can comfort a child in a way that adults and peers often cannot. A pet will listen to a child for hours without interrupting or asking questions. A pet is often content just to be with the child. A pet's antics and playfulness can often engage a child who is emotionally withdrawn. Laughter and tears, hopes and fears can be shared with a pet without the child ever having to feel concerned that his or her feelings may be betrayed or shared with others.

An only child can view a pet as a sibling. The pet might serve as a confidant, a best friend, and a source of comfort and support. This can be especially true of children who are going through a transition such as a move, a divorce, another loss, or an illness.

Children may consider their pets to be protectors, beings who help to keep them safe while the children are sleeping or playing. A pet does not care if a child has a handicap, speech problem, emotional problem, or other disability. Pets love children unconditionally. They do not care if the child got an F on a test or if other children will not play with him or her. A pet is always there for a child, and children come to depend on this source of support and admiration. Pets have a wonderful way of helping children to feel good about themselves.

One client, Liz, who came to the pet loss support group for help in working through the loss of her dog, shared a story about an 11-year-old girl, Sally, and her cat Snowy. Snowy was Sally's best friend. When Sally's parents divorced, Sally relied on Snowy for the love and support she felt she did not receive from her parents, who were absorbed in and overwhelmed by the details of separating.

As Sally and her parents divided their possessions, it was decided that Sally would live with her mother. She and her mother moved into a small house. Liz would visit Sally and her mother frequently. She saw how important Snowy had become to Sally, especially during all of the recent transitions and losses in her life. One night Sally's mother commented to Liz that the cat had fleas and as a result the house was infested with them. She told Liz that she was going to get rid of the cat. Liz told her how much Snowy meant to Sally, encouraged her to allow Sally to keep Snowy, and offered to help her get rid of the fleas. She told the mother what needed to be done to eradicate the fleas. She even offered to come over and assist her in bathing the cat, bombing the house with flea bombs, and then applying flea medication to the cat.

A few weeks later when visiting Sally and her mother, Liz inquired how it was going with Snowy's flea problem. The mother replied that she had limited funds to purchase flea supplies and was feeling too overwhelmed to continue the task of caring for the cat. She told her friend that she had let Snowy go free in a field far from their home. Liz said that she was furious with her friend for letting Snowy go, and felt even more anger over the fact that Sally had seemed to withdraw even further into herself.

Sally was robbed of her chance to say good-bye and of the emotional support she needed to grieve the loss. Her mother treated the cat as an object, one that she had little time or resources to give to, and the relationship her daughter shared with the cat and the importance was disregarded.

This story illustrates how damage can be done to a child who is already suffering when parents fail to realize the important role a pet can play in a child's life.

It is important to note that a child may wonder about or even fear that a parent who can abandon a cherished animal family member (as Snowy was to Sally) might one day abandon the child. Decisions about family pets should not be made in haste. Careful planning and consideration in regard to all family members need to be explored and options need to be discussed.

Caregivers need to bring compassion, warmth, and a desire to understand the child's loss. In his book *Helping Children*

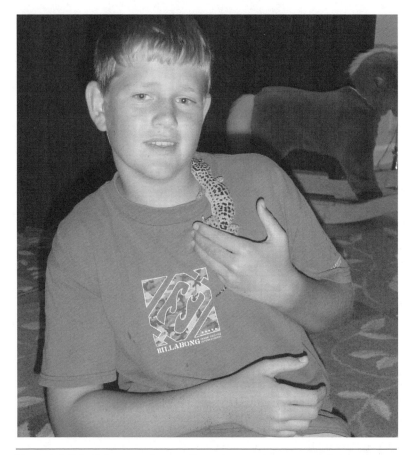

Figure 1.2 Pets that are small or exotic, such as geckos, can nonetheless be very meaningful to the children who love them.

Cope With Grief, Alan Wolfelt outlined a process model for assisting grieving children: "The process contains three important ingredients to develop the desired outcome: The Helper as a Person *plus* The Caring Relationship *plus* Caregiving Skills equals Intended Growth Outcome." The caregiver is an instrument in assisting children through the process of grieving. In assisting children, caregivers must be aware of their life experiences, personal beliefs, strengths and weaknesses of personality, and ways of being in the world. The willingness to look at oneself and how it helps or hinders assisting a grieving child is paramount in helping the child obtain closure and acceptance of the loss. In describing the caregiving relationship, Wolfelt made the point that it must be sensitive to the child, be genuine in warmth, communicate acceptance, and have a true desire to understand the relationship with the pet and depth of the emotion felt by the child. Caregivers must be able to perceive, understand, respond, and effectively express and communicate with the child. Understanding what the pet meant to the child is one of the first steps in helping the child through the loss.[2]

Promoting Healthy Communication Within the Family

The loss of a pet within the family structure should be viewed as a family experience. Some children may experience the death of a classroom pet, and this too can be considered a family experience in the sense that the entire class shared their classroom with the pet and were most likely involved in caring for and interacting with the pet.

Teachers can best assist children through a loss by promoting open communication. One teacher had the children who wanted to participate help to create a classroom mural of the pet and the things the children remembered best. Working on the project opened up a dialogue among the students and with the teacher regarding the loss.

In addition, teachers may want to have a funeral or memorial service for the deceased pet. In cases in which the pet is diagnosed as terminal, the teacher should share this news with the children and allow them to say their good-byes prior to the pet's dying. One idea is that of a good-bye book in which the children draw pictures or write about the feelings they have for the pet either prior to the loss or after it has occurred. Caring for a pet and saying good-bye are lessons in life that offer teachers and caregivers an opportunity to educate and to provide children with knowledge they can use throughout their lifetimes.

Caregivers can share their feelings about the pet and the loss, and encourage children to express their feelings by asking questions, provide honest, age-appropriate answers, and listen to children as they share fears and concerns. Doing these things gives children the support they need to grieve the loss and also helps them build a healthy foundation for future losses.

Effective Communication and Attending Skills

In promoting open communication, caregivers must have good attending skills. Wolfelt wrote, "One of the easiest things to do when communicating with children is to focus so much on what they are saying that you are unaware of the nonverbal messages that your body is sending to them. Your attending and skill many times determines the child's perception of you and your desire and commitment to help. When a difference exists between what you say and what the child reads nonverbally, the nonverbal behavior is always believed as being true. Children are much more sensitive to visual communication than to the spoken word. Nonverbal language is the first language they learn. The way they are held and touched as infants, expression or tone of voice and turn of a head all are elements that have meaning to the small child. From these messages they learn how to understand, make sense of, and respond to their world."[3]

Modeling a child's body posture, sitting cross-legged on the floor, skipping stones side by side, or coloring on a piece of paper are excellent ways of meeting a child at his or her level. The caregiver's body posture is open and nondefensive, and it relates to the child in a way that he or she finds comfortable.

The following example demonstrates how effective open communication and good attending skills can be when working with a grieving child.

Olivia and the READ Program

Olivia was a Portuguese water dog and an extraordinary pet, according to her owner, Sandi Martin, who founded the READ

(Reading Education Assistance Dogs) program. In the READ program, Olivia helped children with reading difficulties by listening patiently as they would read aloud to her. As a therapy dog, she brought comfort, healing, and happiness to many children. Many of the children Olivia and Sandi worked with were challenged physically, emotionally, or developmentally. All the children lacked confidence and possessed low self-esteem; hated performing in front of peers, family, or therapists; and had difficulty focusing on the task at hand. It was often difficult for them to relax. Olivia was a catalyst for change for these children. Olivia's work with children often helped them to improve their reading skills and many advanced two levels or more. The children loved reading to her because she did not laugh at them. She helped them to feel safe as they struggled to learn. Many children stated that they enjoyed reading to Olivia because if they made a mistake she did not care.

One day, Olivia became ill and died. When one of the teachers broke the news about Olivia's death to the students, one 8-year-old boy, Kurt, became very angry. He acted out in class with bad behavior. The teacher approached one of the READ team leaders, John, who had worked with Kurt, and asked him to help. John found Kurt sitting cross-legged on floor near the door outside of the classroom. Kurt appeared to be sullen, and he did not want to talk. When John approached he asked Kurt if he could sit beside him. Kurt shrugged as if he did not care one way or the other. John sat next to Kurt on the floor. After a period of silence John genuinely shared with Kurt that Olivia's death made him sad. Kurt told John that he was angry that Olivia had to die. John said that he could understand Kurt's feelings of anger and that people often feel angry when someone they love dies.

John's acknowledgment of Kurt's feelings allowed Kurt to share further. Kurt shared with John the fact his family had told him not to cry over a pet's dying. John let Kurt know that crying was healthy behavior, and he encouraged him to let his emotions out freely. In sharing his grief, John gave Kurt the validation he so desperately needed for the feelings of loss he was trying to cope with.

Kurt and John attended a memorial service held in Olivia's honor. They and Olivia's friends wrote notes to Olivia that were read at the service and planted a dogwood tree in the school's memory garden. At the memorial, there were 15 huge red balloons attached to the harness of a dog attending the service. At the end of the memorial the balloons were released into the sky, and everyone in attendance thought positive thoughts for Olivia.[4]

Facing Loss

Parents need to confront their own feelings about death and dying before being able to help their child through a loss. Grieving a loss is painful and hard work. Parents might find that they have unresolved feelings about past losses. They might remember earlier losses of their own pets and how their parents dealt with them. There might be some unresolved feelings regarding past losses. The more parents work through their own feelings regarding loss, the better they will be able to help their child through one. Caregivers who have difficulty with their feelings regarding loss will benefit from seeking professional support.

It is important to remember that with each new loss we are given an opportunity to work through previous losses. This opportunity is presented to both children and adults. Many adults have unresolved issues regarding the loss of childhood pets and other human losses. As I mentioned, past losses can involve other people and animals. But they also can involve losing attachment objects and habits (e.g., pacifiers, blankets, nursing) and learning that there is no Santa Claus, Easter Bunny, or Tooth Fairy. One mother told me that when her daughter learned that these things were not "real," she questioned the existence of God and felt betrayed by her mother's "lies" about these mythical characters she had believed in for the first 10 years of her life. This crisis of faith this was also an opportunity for the child and her mother to work through the loss. This was a time for her daughter to learn more about why her mother chose to help create the magical illusion of Santa Claus for her daughter and to discuss the importance of the spirit of Christmas and the faith their family practiced. This topic has been beautifully written about by Valentine Davies in *Miracle on 34th Street,* which was made into a classic film. Addressing a crisis of faith, Davies wrote, "Faith is believing in things when common sense tells you not to."[5] In working through loss, it is vital that children be encouraged to have faith.

Children and adults need to believe that the pain of a loss will pass and that joy will once again be experienced in life. Children need to know that their feelings are acknowledged and shared and that grieving can be done with support and is not something that must be faced alone.

Caregivers must realize that sharing feelings with a child is healthy. If a child shares, "I feel so angry that Sugar died, Mommy," the parent might say, "It's okay to feel angry about Sugar dying. Sometimes I feel angry about it too." The only time a parent may want to consider minimizing the depth of feeling being expressed is when the child feels burdened by it.

Children are often sensitive and compassionate to those around them. If the child expresses fears about the depth of feeling being expressed by an adult, the adult should seek outside support for himself or herself. On the other hand, not sharing feelings of grief with a child by being "strong" for a child does not allow the child to learn how grief is dealt with and worked through. It is vital for the child's mental health to learn how to express feelings and to receive answers to his or her questions.

Many of us wish that we had the right words at the right time. Unfortunately, this is not always possible. However, there are guidelines to keep in mind when helping a child who is experiencing a loss.

Caregiver Dos and Don'ts

Do say the following:

- I'm sorry.
- I cannot imagine how difficult this must be for you.
- How are you feeling?
- I don't know what to say. (If this is the case.)
- I'd like to hear about your feelings.
- I care about you.
- We have a lot of memories together regarding [pet]. Do you remember when . . . ?
- Tell me about your pet.

Do not say the following:

- At least you have other pets.
- You can get another pet to replace the one you lost.
- God needed him more than you did.
- Your pet is in a better place.
- It was God's will.
- I know just how you feel.
- It was just a pet.
- Don't cry.
- You should . . .
- You shouldn't . . .
- You have to be strong.
- Big boys [or girls] don't cry.

Know that there is nothing you can say to make it all better for the child. Acknowledging the loss and validating the depth of the feelings experienced are first steps in assisting a child. One of the most painful experiences a caregiver can have is to watch a child suffer. It is natural to want to fix it, to make it right. With loss, however, it takes time to work through feelings. Poet Robert Frost wrote, "The best way out is always through." Children must go through the process of grief to resolve their feelings and live their lives to the fullest.

To encourage a child to unfold his or her feelings, caregivers should be good listeners, which involves being in close proximity to the grieving child. Create a safe environment for the child to discuss his or her feelings. Make the environment warm, friendly, and inviting by being warm, friendly, and open. Younger children may discuss their feelings while drawing or playing with building blocks with you. Older children may decide to open up during a car ride. This is a good time to keep the radio turned off or down low.

Do not judge, blame, or shame the child when he or she is talking about the loss or impending loss. Do not rush in with comments or questions. Just listen and respond thoughtfully and intuitively. Do not diminish the depth of feeling being expressed by the child. Avoid phrases such as, "Oh, it isn't that bad." Let the child tell you how he or she feels. If the child is sharing feelings and crying, acknowledge the sadness he or she is feeling. You might say, "We feel sad when a pet that we have loved dies." Use accurate language when talking about the pet's death. Refer to the pet as being dead, not as having been lost or having passed on. If you deny the reality of the death, the grieving child might feel as if he or she has to please you by denying the pet's death. Remember that it is normal for children to bring up the loss over and over again. As the child matures, so will his or her understanding of the pet's death.

Children often know intuitively when things are not right or when they are being lied to. Taking cues from adults and using careful observation, children often draw conclusions about what is going on around them. If the caregivers do not deal with their own grief over the loss of a pet, then children learn that it is bad or wrong to discuss feelings or display emotions. It is important for children to see that when a loss occurs, a period of mourning follows.

In 1969, Dr. Elisabeth Kubler-Ross outlined five predictable stages of grief in her book *On Death and Dying*.[6] These stages are routinely used to describe the levels of grief children and adults experience when a loss occurs. In this book I include six stages: denial, bargaining, anger, guilt, sorrow, and resolution. Guilt is not so much a separate stage as it is a pervasive entity that crosses all phases and can hinder progress from one stage to the next. The grief process is not a steady, linear ascent from sadness to joy. It is like a roller coaster ride with ups and downs at every turn. At the end of the ride is a place of acceptance and resolution, where the child comes to terms with the loss and is at peace. It is the job of the therapist to facilitate a smooth transition from one stage to the next and to help children move as quickly as possible out of phases in which they become stuck. A skilled therapist will recognize all aspects of grief, including hidden ones.[7]

Recognizing Hidden Grief

Children may not always show immediate grief. They may internalize their feelings and express them through acts of aggression, verbal or physical. We see this in play therapy. A child who cannot or will not articulate his or her feelings will often be willing to act them out through play. It is safer to play a role, to hide behind a toy, and to disguise feelings if children are not sure that they will be accepted, validated, or understood by adults.

There are two kinds of hidden grief we look at in this chapter. One kind of grief is a chosen hidden grief and involves grief feelings the child chooses not to share with a caregiver. This type of grief, the result of a conscious decision to hide grief, is poignantly illustrated in the film *In America*. The other kind of grief is best described as unaware hidden grief. This type of grief is hidden to the child.

Chosen Hidden Grief

A child's grieving may get "lost" or be dismissed by parents who are too absorbed in dealing with their own grief. Sometimes children keep their grief hidden from their parents in order to protect them. In the film *In America,* the oldest daughter, the preteenage Christy, makes a powerful statement to her father regarding the death of her little brother Frankie: "I've been carrying this family for two years!" She explains to her father that her mother had been too overcome with the grief of losing "her son" and he at losing "his son" to notice that she too was in pain. Christy said that Frankie was "*her* brother" and that she had endured a tremendous loss as well. Christy says, "I cried too, and I talked to Frankie every night until one night I realized I was talking to myself."[8]

Christy chose not to burden her parents with her grief while they were working through the loss of their son. She took on the role of protecting the adults who should have been caring for her, and, as a result, she suffered greatly.

Other children may not even be aware of the depth of their emotion experienced when a loss occurs. This type of grief is hidden from the child.

Unaware Hidden Grief

Children are often unaware of deeper feelings that arise from a death and lack understanding about how to integrate them into the process of grieving.

One example of hidden grief was experienced by a parent who thought that her 9-year-old daughter was handling a recent move and the loss of her cat well. Her daughter, Carissa, seemed to take everything in stride. Carissa received very high marks in school on her report card and Carissa's teacher said that Carissa behaved wonderfully in the classroom. Soon after, Carissa and her younger brother were fighting over a video game at home. Carissa had decided that they each would play the game for 10 minutes and then switch. When the younger sibling refused to switch, Carissa pushed him away from the game. The mother intervened and told Carissa to stop playing. When she refused, the mother took the game away from her daughter. Carissa became angrier and spit at her mom. Her mom was shocked and hurt by Carissa's behavior.

The next day Carissa told her mother that she was going out to play. When her mother told her that she had to finish her homework first, Carissa told her she was going anyway. When the mother walked over to say absolutely not, Carissa kicked her in the shin.

Several days later, after meeting with a therapist, Carissa told her mother that she was very angry with her for not allowing her to say good-bye to her dying cat. The mother apologized to Carissa and told her that she had not realized that it was so important to Carissa to say good-bye before the cat went to the veterinarian to be euthanized.

She and Carissa talked through the hurt and angry feelings. The therapist told Carissa and her mom that this was an opportunity to learn how to safely express anger. They discussed ways in which Carissa could write out her feelings or draw them. They also came up with a way for Carissa to say good-bye to her cat. They held a memorial service, and Carissa wrote a letter to the cat and read it at the service.

Sometimes children do not even realize that they are feeling anger or sadness over a loss. They may become temporarily preoccupied or purposely busy themselves. Eventually feelings that accompany grief and loss will occur. These feelings may come out in response to a daily event, and may be carried to an extreme (as in the example of Carissa and her mother). Children often show their feelings to those with whom they are closest. In this example, Carissa felt safe expressing her anger to her mother.

Other children may say that they never liked the pet anyway and that they are glad that it is dead or missing. This might be a way of expressing anger at the pet for abandoning them. They may withdraw from other people or pets that they love out of fear of being hurt again. Sometimes parents try to downplay or minimize the grief experience for the child by choosing not to talk about it or acting as if it did not happen. If adults treat the loss as insignificant, children may fear that if something were to happen to them, the adults would not care.

Whenever there is a loss, many different feelings are involved. Because of this, there is tremendous opportunity for human development when a loss occurs. Although it can be frightening to witness or receive the brunt of a child's deep feelings, adults should realize that they have been given an opportunity to help the child grow successfully toward autonomy. Therapists can assist parents and caregivers by giving them the tools they might need to work at home with the child. Discussing appropriate ways in which to express anger, say things that acknowledge and validate feelings, and listen effectively can assist a caregiver in keeping an open, healthy, and close relationship with a child.

Another example of unaware hidden grief is illustrated in the case example of Emily and Harvey.

Emily and Harvey   According to her mother, 9-year-old Emily's best friend was her cat Harvey. Harvey disappeared one day. He was discovered hiding under the front porch of their house several days later. He was injured. The veterinarian who examined Harvey gave a poor prognosis for recovery. The only treatment available would be extensive and costly.

Harvey was given less than a 10% chance of recovery. The family discussed the options and included Emily in the discussion. Emily's mother said that she could not afford the costly treatment. She was concerned that even if she could find a way to pay for it, Harvey would experience a great deal of misery with little hope of recovery. Emily said that she wanted Harvey to live. Her mother explained to her how Harvey would suffer if they chose to treat him. In the end, Emily and her mother opted to euthanize Harvey.

Emily was permitted to say her final good-byes to Harvey at the veterinarian's office. A few weeks after Harvey's death, Emily still cried intermittently. She had difficulty concentrating in school and chose to remain at home instead of playing with her friends. Emily's mother sought the help of a therapist when Emily's appetite diminished and her sleep was disturbed.

Emily finally shared with the therapist her fear that if she became seriously injured or ill, her mother would not be able to afford treatment for her. Emily's fears were resolved when her mother reassured Emily that Emily was her first priority. Emily's mother said that she would always make certain she could adequately provide for her daughter. She reminded Emily that she had loved Harvey too. She told Emily that although financial considerations were a factor in making the decision, a more important factor was the suffering Harvey would have endured if they had not chosen euthanasia.

Emily was able to accept this new information and resume her normal activities. She and her mother found ways to memorialize Harvey: Emily named a favorite stuffed animal after him, and she and her mother created a collage from their favorite photos of Harvey. They held a ceremony at Harvey's grave site.

Emily had a best-friend relationship with Harvey. In understanding how children are affected by pet loss, we need to have specific information on the level of importance and meaning the pet had in the child's life. Emily's mother was able to fill in the emotional gaps that Harvey's death left for Emily. She became Emily's friend and confidant by validating the importance and significance of Emily's loss. She demonstrated the depth of her feelings for Emily by acknowledging the loss and finding ways in which she could assist Emily in coping with it. More important, once the therapist informed the mother of Emily's fears, her mother communicated effectively with Emily, thus reassuring her.[9]

Caregivers must be receptive to all of the feelings that accompany a loss. Children should be allowed to express their anger, fears, grief, concerns, and heartfelt emotions.

Linda Goldman, in her book *Breaking the Silence,* wrote that caregivers sometimes perceive a child's need to discuss the details of a loss as manipulative.[10] They may tell the child not to talk about the death or feelings surrounding it. Children need to talk about what happened to make sense of the loss and work through it.

Children can effectively work through their fears by using the following techniques.. They can also draw a picture of their fears. Ask the children if they have any secrets about the loss. If they do not want to say them out loud, they can write them in a journal or on a piece of paper or even whisper them to a favorite toy. The children can decide if and when they want to share them. Writing down the fear allows children to let it out. Children's choosing to share the fear with a trusted caregiver enables the caregiver to dispel the fear.

Once a fear is out in the open, the caregiver can assist the child in working through the fear. Providing children with factual information can help to dispel many fears. Sometimes children fear that they may have caused the pet's demise.

Conclusion

As caregivers, we must understand what the pets mean to children to effectively assist them through a loss. This is best achieved by asking the children about the pet. How children experience the relationship shared with the pet determines the level of grief they will feel with the loss of a pet. Understanding the relationship children share with pets is the first step in helping them to work through a loss.

Therapists should encourage parents to face their own feelings regarding the death of the pet to effectively assist their children. When parents have unresolved issues involving loss, the issues can get in the way of helping their children. Parents may need support in learning how much information is appropriate to share with their children regarding the death of a pet and in encouraging their children to share their own feelings.

Children may have hidden grief. They may choose to protect their parents from their grief by not expressing their feelings or not talking about the loss with them. They may be unaware of their feelings and deepest fears regarding death and dying and not know how to express them.

Pet loss is a family experience in which each member's grief needs to be validated and worked through. Sharing feelings of grief and loss promotes healthy communication and can work to bring a family closer together.

2
How Children Assimilate Loss

Strange is our situation here upon earth. Each of us comes for a short visit, not knowing why, yet sometimes seeming to divine purpose. From the standpoint of daily life, however, there is one thing we do know: That we are here for the sake of others . . . for the countless unknown souls with whose fate we are connected by a bond of sympathy. Many times a day, I realize how much my own outer and inner life is built upon the labors of people, both living and dead, and how earnestly I must exert myself in order to give in return as much as I have received.

—Albert Einstein

It is human nature to try to find meaning and purpose in life. From the time that we are very young, we question why things are the way that they are. Why do animals and people we love die? Cultural and spiritual beliefs vary greatly in our society. Although it is important to share our personal beliefs with our own children and to respect the beliefs of families with whom we work, it remains true that children will go through similar stages of grief. We feel sadness when someone we love dies. Supporting a grieving child through the loss of a pet can send a powerful message to the child. Not only does it acknowledge the bond shared with the pet and the depth and meaning of that bond for the child, it relays

21

to the child that expressing grief is healthy, an expected part of life. In addition, it lets the child know that by grieving he or she is honoring the life that was shared with the pet.

In acknowledging the bond and the depth of feeling that accompanies this loss, we teach the child that he or she matters and is also cared for deeply. Often in life, it is in the struggle that we learn the most about ourselves. Through addressing our grief consciously, we derive a sense of inner strength, true empathy, and compassion not only for our own process but also for that of others who are also grieving. This is one of the most significant developments in the life of a child for building a strong sense of self and a feeling of belonging in the world.

The Process of Grieving and Self-Esteem

When we look at loss, the process of grieving, and how they directly affect self-esteem, the importance of establishing a healthy foundation for grief takes on a new significance. How the child perceives the loss and the support or lack of support he or she receives while going through the grieving process will help to shape his or her view of self and of others.

Psychologist Carl Rogers stated in *Client Centered Therapy*, "As experiences occur in the life of the individual, they are either (a) symbolized, perceived, and organized into some relationship to the self, (b) ignored because there is no perceived relationship to the self-structure, or (c) denied symbolization or given a distorted symbolization because the experience is inconsistent with the structure of the self."[1]

Most of the ways of behaving that are adopted by the individual are those that are consistent with the concept of self. From Rogers's propositions, one can conclude that how a child perceives a loss can have an effect on how the child views himself or herself. For example, if the child is made to believe (through words, actions, or lack of action) that the loss of a beloved pet is meaningless (e.g., an authority figure saying to a grieving child who shared significant feelings for his pet cat, "Don't be sad over the loss of the cat, we can get another one"), he may come to view himself as having little or no value to others. Likewise, Rogers said, "When the individual perceives and accepts into one consistent and integrated system all his sensory and visceral experiences, then he is necessarily more understanding of others and is more accepting of others as separate individuals."[2]

Trust, autonomy, and identity are the basis of the foundation for healthy development in children. Levy and Orlans further explained this by stating that "trust develops during the first-year-of-life attachment cycle: Need, arousal, gratification and trust. The baby learns to trust caregivers (reliable and sensitive; will meet my needs); self (my needs are acceptable; I am worthwhile); and the external world (I feel safe and protected, my world is okay). The development of basic trust is a primary development task of the first year of life and serves as a foundation for future emotional and social growth."[3]

Although pet loss is often one of the first losses experienced by children, it is important to recognize that we start experiencing feelings of loss from the time we are infants. Children must learn to sleep alone and to give up nursing, diapers, bottles, pacifiers, and various love objects. When a beloved toy or blanket is lost, our first inclination might be to replace the object to minimize or prevent grief in the child. However, to the child, the lost object might be irreplaceable. Although feelings of love, comfort, and being needed derived from the object may be transferred to another object, the one that is lost can never be replaced. Often, a child experiences a sense of sadness or anxiety over the loss even if what has been lost is not a living being.

It is important to support children in their quest for autonomy while being sensitive to their losses. We must look at the children's point of view and be supportive, nurturing, and empathetic to help them grow and develop without getting stuck in the process of grieving. If we can do this, we are helping children to grow into adults with the necessary skills for maintaining mentally healthy lives.

To provide the type of support a grieving child needs, we must first understand how children of varying developmental stages assimilate loss. But regardless of children's ages, a trusted adult's openness and honesty will encourage children to ask questions about death and loss that will enable them to work through their experiences. Sometimes children will ask their questions immediately, but it is not uncommon for questions to surface over several years as children mature and their levels of awareness increase.

Some mental health experts feel that children are not mature enough to work through a deeply felt loss until they are adolescents. Children are likely to express their sadness on and off over many years, and in indirect ways. Being able to continue exploring death and loss while maturing helps the child build a strong foundation for working through losses as an adult. This is especially true when a deeply felt pet loss occurs, because many people can be more supportive of the loss of a parent or sibling and because the emotion felt can be viewed as less significant than emotions associated with human losses.

As children mature, their knowledge expands. They need to integrate what they learn about death with the rest of their knowledge about the world. Although it can be painful for an adult to have the loss brought up repeatedly, it is important to remember that children need a long time to work through a loss. A useful analogy is to compare the process of guiding children through grief with the process of building a sturdy structure that will stand strong for many years to come.[4]

Isabelle and Lady

An 85-year-old woman, Isabelle, whom I met at the pet loss support group I lead, was sharing her feelings of sadness over the recent loss of her dog Lady. Although Isabelle remembered the life she had shared with Lady, she recalled many of the other losses she endured throughout her lifetime. She shared with the group a story about how her mother had explained death to her when Isabelle was 7 years old and they were living in England: "I had heard older people talking about illness and dying. I went to my mother and asked my mother if it hurt to die. She didn't say yes and she didn't say no. She just took me by the hand and led me out to the garden. She told me to look around at all the beautiful flowers in the garden. 'Do you see how lovely the flowers are now, Isabelle?' I said, 'Yes, Mama.' She then told me that soon the flowers would wither and die in the fall. But in the spring, she said, the flowers would bloom again and new ones would grow. 'That is how death is, Isabelle.' I never forgot that lesson."

Isabelle was able to embrace that definition of loss and apply it throughout her life. She loved and lost many people (including a husband in World War II) and numerous pets. Perhaps for her, trusting in loving another person or pet again corresponded with her trust in the flowers in the garden, which her mother showed her would bloom again.

A Pet Is a Family Responsibility

Sometimes adults are surprised at the intensity of a child's grief. They may comment that the child did not seem as interested in the pet when it was alive as he or she does now that it has died. When children are seeking their own identities, they can go through periods of distancing themselves from pets, as they do with other family members. Also, a child might distance himself or herself from an ill or dying pet. It should not be assumed that the child did not care deeply for the pet. Most important, an adult should never make a child feel guilty because he or she did not seem to care for the pet prior to the loss. One 7-year-old boy needed to talk a lot about whether his pet cockatiel Pumpkin escaped and flew away because he had forgotten to latch the cage door properly, as his mother had admonished him. The therapist helped the child work through his feelings regarding the loss of his bird by having him draw a picture of Pumpkin and talk about it. Although supporting the child in accepting the reality of what had happened and the role he may have played in the loss, the therapist also let the child know that a pet is the responsibility of the entire family. Children need to have support for the feelings they are experiencing in the moment.

Children whose parents give a pet away because they believe the children were not taking enough responsibility for the pet's care will need particular understanding in fully working through any feelings of guilt associated with the loss of the pet. Parents should be encouraged to explain to a child that the pet needed to have a home where he could be cared for on a regular basis. Children should be allowed and encouraged to say good-bye to their pets. If possible, they should be able to visit their pet in its new home. Deciding to adopt and care for a pet should be a family decision. I cannot stress this fact enough: All family members should share in the responsibility for the pet's care. Children whose pets are not well cared for should not be blamed for the pets' demise or be shamed in any way. When adopting a pet, children can be told what is expected of them regarding its care.

Expectations should be age appropriate. Ultimately, the parents are responsible for the pet's well-being, which involves making certain that the children follow through in caring for the pet. Have a pet should be a positive learning experience. When expectations are exceeding the child's abilities, tragic loss of the pet can occur and feelings of worthlessness, guilt, and anger can arise in the child.

One parent, who adopted a young rabbit for her 5-year-old daughter, discovered that taking care of a pet involved more care than she expected when she had first accepted the responsibility for the pet. The parent had thought that the child was ready to help with the care of the pet but soon discovered that this was not the case. A decision was made to place the rabbit in another home. The parent asked the new adoptive family if her daughter could come see the pet in its new home.

The family agreed. The daughter was able to say good-bye to her pet rabbit and see it in its new home, which assisted her through a transition period in which her bond with her rabbit was honored. The fact that the parents shared in the responsibility of acknowledging that the family needed to place the rabbit in a new home was also helpful.

The parents told their daughter that the decision to let another family adopt the pet, although involving some sadness and difficulty, was made out of love for the pet and that they might try again, in the future, to adopt another pet.

It is not uncommon for children who do not have brothers and sisters to perceive a pet as a best friend, confidant, or sibling. Caregivers working with children of any age should know that it is important to learn what the pet meant to that child. Direct questioning in regard to the relationship might work with older children, such as "How do you feel about the loss of your dog?" However, with younger children, allowing the child to articulate it or re-create the relationship through symbols (e.g., art therapy) might reveal more.

Spiritual Beliefs and Religious Convictions

For therapists assisting a child through a pet loss, it is important to ask the parents about any religious beliefs the family holds. This will help the therapist to support and respect the family's beliefs about death, dying, and the hereafter, even if they do not share those beliefs. In building rapport with a therapist, a child may question the therapist about his or her beliefs. It is important to be honest and forthright with a child. However, the discussion can be genuine but brief; lengthy explanations are not always necessary, especially for very young children. For example, if a therapist who practices Catholicism is questioned by a child whose family practices Buddhism about whether the therapist believes that the deceased pet will be reincarnated, the therapist could briefly say, "I know that is a belief that you and your family share and I respect your beliefs." If questioned further, the therapist might choose to share that he or she does not practice Buddhism but appreciates the fact that the child and his or her family do. The important thing is to be honest, open, and genuine and to reflect back to the child the core sense of what you feel he or she is attempting to understand.

In his book *Talking About Death: A Dialogue Between Parent and Child,* Earl Grollman suggested that parents not express any religious convictions they do not actually hold. Children will detect the inconsistency and deception in a tale about heavenly happiness when they see their parents struggling with feelings of hopelessness, finality, and despair. Painting too beautiful a picture of the hereafter can even entice a child to wanting to join the pet in heaven. Telling children that God took Mittens because he was special and good can frighten children. They may fear that if they are too good, God might decide to take them as well. Grollman encouraged parents to share only honestly felt religious convictions that they are willing to explain to their children. One example is that of a 5-year-old girl who began to behave badly at home after her dog died. She often did the opposite of what her mother asked her to do. Her mother was at a loss as how to handle her daughter's behavior when she asked the therapist to meet with her.

After a few play therapy sessions with the therapist, the little girl shared with her that she did not want to die. The therapist asked her why she thought she might die. She told her that her dog had gone to heaven because he was very good. The therapist learned that the girl's grandmother had told the little girl that God took the dog to be with him in heaven because he was such a good dog. Once the little girl learned that her grandmother had said this to her to comfort her and that her dog died because he had a sickness that the doctors were not able to cure, the little girl returned to her normal behavior.

Cognitive Age and Effects of Loss

In working with children, especially very young children, caregivers might find it difficult to find the right words. If told that a pet died because it was sick, a child might fear that when he is sick he might die. If told that a dead pet is sleeping, a child might fear that the pet will wake up after it is buried. Caregivers must think very carefully before they speak. If something is misunderstood or stated in a way that the child might misinterpret, it should be clarified at the time. If a caregiver does not know the answer to a child's question, the caregiver should tell the child that he or she does not know. If appropriate, the caregiver can discuss how to find out the answer.

How much can children understand about an emotionally felt loss and what should they be told about it? If we are old enough to feel love, then we can feel a loss when that love being expressed to us is gone. A child's level of cognitive development directly correlates with the effects of loss the child experiences. Based loosely on Piaget's stages of development, the following outline illustrates what grief reactions can be expected from children of varying ages.[5]

Birth to age 2 years. Studies have shown that even infants can experience stress, resulting in feelings of isolation and abandonment. Infants can sense when there is discord in their environment. They can react by crying, clinging, being difficult to console, withdrawing, sleeping too much or too little, or regressing to previous behaviors. Children of this age can be reassured through touching, hugging, holding, and rocking. Speaking to them in a soothing voice also helps reduce anxiety during times of stress and loss.

Ages 2 years to 5 years. A young child's ability to understand and use information about what is happening in the immediate surroundings should not be underestimated. Children should be told what has happened to their pet and why.

As the child matures, pet loss can be linked to imaginative play. Preschoolers might hold a funeral service, or they might think of the pet as alive in some other place, such as heaven. They might believe that when a pet dies it is only asleep and will one day awaken, or they might ask how the pet will be able to return to them after being buried in the ground. Too often their belief that the pet is only sleeping is reinforced when we use the common euphemism for euthanasia, saying the pet was "put to sleep." A child might bury a dead animal, then dig it up a few days later to see what is happening to it. Children this age need help in understanding the finality of a pet's death. They need to be told that the pet is not sleeping and will not be able to return home.

The most severe symptoms of distress appear in children who are not informed about their pets' fates. Symptomatic distress behaviors in a child this age include hitting, biting, kicking, disobeying, regressing to previous behaviors (e.g., sucking a thumb, refusing to use the toilet, showing increased need for transitional objects), throwing temper tantrums, withdrawing, masturbating, and exhibiting separation anxiety. The child might have nightmares or psychosomatic symptoms (e.g., stomachaches, preoccupation with small hurts). The child may or may not display immediate signs of grief.

Children this age need encouragement to work through their feelings. Dramatic play, drawing, or talking about the loss often helps. Play therapy (which we explore in more depth in chapter 4) can be very beneficial for a child working through a loss. Children should be encouraged to ask questions and receive honest answers. They may need reassurance that their parents are not leaving them and are available to provide them with the love and support they need.

Ages 6 years to 11 years. When children are 6 years old and older, they are able to view death as the final stage of life. They know that the pet is gone and is not coming back. However, many children this age might believe that death is something that happens only to others or see it as a punishment for having done something bad. They might rationalize that the pet died because it was bad or because the child was bad, or because the child's angry thoughts killed it.

Children can show signs of grief sporadically. They can feel angry at the pet for dying and say that they never wanted it and are glad that it is gone. These children need encouragement in working through their feelings. They might find it therapeutic to write a letter to the pet, draw pictures, or use some other form of self-expression. Many children have worked through angry feelings by keeping a journal. What is written in the journal should be kept private and shared with a caregiver only if the child so desires. It is important to allow children the space and privacy they need to fully work through their feelings. School and interactions with peers can be positive factors during a loss. Often, children feel better if they are allowed to continue with their same routines and friendships. Activity at school can be a positive distraction for the child, much like an adult's work.

Danny and Raticus

One parent described the loss of a 2-year-old pet rat Raticus, who was loved dearly by her 10-year-old son Danny: "We had a lot tears when she was dying. When the time came to euthanize Raticus, Danny told me that he didn't want to be a part of the euthanasia, he just wanted me to take care of it while he was at school. He said that he didn't want to talk about it when he got home and that he wanted the cage and things that belonged with the rat removed from his room. I honored his wishes." He also told his mom that it "hurt too bad" to lose a pet and that he never wanted another one. His mom acknowledged the pain that comes from losing something we love. She told him that although she understood that right now he never wanted to give his heart to another animal again, in time he might decide to, and either way was OK.

It was several months later that Danny approached his mom about possibly adopting another rat. He wondered if it would be a betrayal to Raticus to love another pet. His mom explained to him that adopting another rat would not be a betrayal of the life he shared with Raticus, and that it was OK to want to give his love to another pet. She said that when he was ready they could look for another rat. She explained to Danny that he might bond with the first rat he saw, or it might take a while to find just the right friend, but that he would know when he met the rat. Eventually, Danny chose to adopt another pet rat.

This example of Danny and Raticus illustrates open communication with the parent and respect of feelings regarding the loss, which enabled Danny to fully work through his feelings. Children who do not receive the support they need might exhibit other behaviors during the grieving period. Children this age can express their fears through depression, aggression, dependency, phobias, compulsive eating, and feelings of rejection, denial, and anxiety.

Meaning of Loss

Children might ask questions about the meaning of a loss. They might want to know where, if anywhere, the pet's spirit has gone. They may need to have death explained to them and to be allowed to express what they believe happens spiritually, if anything. This is often a good time for parents to discuss spiritual and religious beliefs with children. Poetry, literature, dance, drama, and films such as *Old Yeller* can provide some comfort to a grieving child. Some literary examples include *When a Pet Dies, All Dogs Go to Heaven,* and *The Tenth Good Thing About Barney* (see chapter 10).

Marty Tousley, R.N., wrote in her booklet *Children and Pet Loss: A Guide for Helping,* "Like all of us, children need to learn that death and loss are natural parts of living. We know that nothing in life lasts forever. Every living thing goes through a natural process with a beginning and an ending, with living in between."[6] The following story, one of the most poignant explanations of death I have ever heard, illustrates this philosophy.

This vignette took place in the classic film starring Sophia Loren and Cary Grant, *Houseboat*.[7] A young boy is angry over the loss of his mother. He tells his father that dead is dead and that he does not believe in anything anymore. Grant's character says, "I prefer to think that no one ever really leaves." His father then explains his own beliefs about loss by using a pitcher of water. He explains that the pitcher is a container that holds water, much like a person's body is a container that holds the soul. The water represents the persons' life force. He then pours the water onto the deck of the boat, and he and his son watch as the water rolls off the deck into the lake. He tells his son that the water, without the pitcher, is still water. The son says, "Oh, I get it." He then says to his dad that the water flows into the lake, goes back up into the clouds, and eventually becomes rain. Through this metaphor, Grant's character lets his son know that he believes the essence or spirit of his mother, even without her body, will always be with them. Grant's character says, "Everything is always changing," and he continues to explain, "I believe when our life force leaves our body we go back into God's universe and our life force goes back into nature and becomes a part of everything that we know. That sort of change [is] very beautiful."

Through this illustration, a father teaches his son that his mother lives on in everything that is a part of life and that they will continue to love and remember her. I chose this illustration to demonstrate that when working with children through a loss, we need to be honest with ourselves, honest with them, open to listening and discussing, and perhaps creative in expressing what we believe so that the children can understand.

Helping children to find hope, especially during a loss, can give them something to hold onto during a difficult time. They can be reminded to look for the rainbow after the storm and to have faith that sad, angry, and lonely feelings accompanying the loss will subside and feelings of joy in remembering the life shared with the pet will return. It can also make a significant difference in how children view the rest of life's losses.

Cognitive Age and Loss in the Teen Years

Ages 12 years to 17 years. Children in this age group might ask questions about what would happen to them if their parents were to die. These children's feelings need to be acknowledged and validated. They need to be reassured that plans have been made for this eventuality and that they will be lovingly provided for if this happens. In addition, they need to be told that the vast majority of people live for a long time. Because individuation is a major task of the developing child during adolescence, children should be allowed to have input into the decision-making processes about their lives and about their pets. They should be encouraged to develop a healthy balance of dependence and independence.

The loss of a pet can remind children of a previous loss they experienced that they might not have worked through. They might ask questions about the past loss. Some of these questions might require philosophical answers. Children this age also might ask about disposal of the pet's body. Truthful information will help to lessen the child's anxiety about the loss. Children are the best guides in letting others know how much information they need.

As children enter their teen years, they begin their search for the meaning of life. They want to know how to cope with loss. It is important to make certain that they have the tools they need to work through a loss successfully and fully. A child who has endured other losses—such as a move, a change of schools, the loss of friendships, or divorce—might have viewed a pet as a source of comfort throughout childhood. When the bond between the child and pet is broken, the child may not know how to handle difficult situations without the comforting presence of that pet. This should alert the therapist that there is a lack of support within the family structure. The child may have learned to rely on the pet for emotional support during times when the parents were not available. This is an opportunity for the parent to learn to help the child and provide the child with the emotional support needed to work through a loss.

I remember when we moved from Michigan to Minnesota when I was 12 years old. My pets were two goldfish. My parents wanted me to give the fish away prior to the move. However, I refused, and pleaded with them to let them move with us. My parents relented. As we drove through Michigan, Wisconsin, and then through Minnesota, those two fish rode on my lap in their little bowl. To my parents' credit, they understood that not only was I bonded to the fish but the fish also reminded me of the home and friends I was leaving behind. They helped me to transition into a new environment and to make new friends.

Children might become depressed during a loss or while anticipating a loss. Children may experience anxiety, eat too much or too little, have difficulty sleeping or concentrating, or refuse to participate in things they once enjoyed. Depressive symptoms in children of this age can include thoughts of suicide. Any mention of suicide should be taken seriously. Children exhibiting these symptoms should be promptly assessed for depression and treated by a medical doctor (this topic is explored in depth in chapter 7).

Children need to have their feelings validated and to learn ways to cope with loss. Interactions with peers who have experienced a similar loss can be helpful. Children this age are able to empathize genuinely with and support each other. Although children should be encouraged to express feelings of grief openly, it is just as important to let them know that it is all right to enjoy themselves, too. Children, like adults, should be able to take a break from painful reminders of a pet's passing. Taking time to play and enjoy friends or sports activities should be encouraged if the child so desires. It is important for children to know that it is healthy to do things that bring them joy and that their pets would want them to go on living their lives to the fullest.

In preparing her 11-year-old son Trevor for the death of his terminally ill pet rat Daisy, the mother continually reminded Trevor to enjoy the time that he and Daisy had left together. One day Trevor blurted out to his mother, "I just want you to stop talking about it!" In talking more about the impending loss, Trevor expressed that he did not want to be continually reminded, that he wanted to enjoy being with her without thinking about when she was going to die. A better way to talk to a child about an impending loss is to talk to the child truthfully about what is happening (e.g., "Daisy is very old and very sick. She will not live much longer.") and to remind the child about the things he did well in taking care of the pet (e.g., "I like how you talk to Daisy and how gentle you are when handling her. She is well loved by you."). Comments such as these will assist the child by acknowledging the bond he feels for the pet and help him to view himself as a good pet owner. The important thing to remember when talking to a child is to be genuine in your comments.

Pet Loss in Adulthood

Older than age 18 years. If an adult had a healthy experience with loss as a child, he or she will possess the cognitive and emotional abilities to understand death and loss throughout his or her life. Adults continue to look for meaning in life and death. Healthy adults have the ability to reason, to seek help when needed, and to handle difficult situations such as death and loss.

Young adults may have to leave their pets with their parents or find suitable homes for them when moving to another

location (e.g., leaving for college). Saying good-bye to a beloved pet can be difficult. Many young adults describe leaving
a pet as closing a chapter on their childhood. An older adult
can help a person this age recognize that he or she may be
grieving not only the loss of a pet but also the loss of childhood.

I often work with people who have had horses throughout
their childhoods. Horse owners can have a horse for 20 years
or more, starting in childhood and lasting into adulthood.
When a horse dies, not only is that bond broken but also a
significant tie to the past is gone, which is similar to when an
adult loses a parent.

Conclusion

If we are to be effective in working with children through
loss, we must be patient and willing to listen and learn what
the loss means to them. As the child matures, his or her understanding of the loss also deepens. Children might continue
to ask questions about a loss that occurred years before. They
may use this opportunity to question unresolved issues of
loss in other areas of their lives, such as divorce, moves, or
changes in schools.

Understanding the cognitive stages of development can help
us to assist children through a loss. I often let people know
that death education is not unlike sex education, in that the
child's cognitive stage of development is one of the best indicators of how much information the child needs and can ab-
sorb. It is also similar in that children will often ask what
they need to know and no further explanation is necessary
at the time. As a child matures and develops he or she may
further question the loss and want more information.

If children feel safe and free to openly seek out what they
need to know, they will be laying a sturdy foundation on which
to build through future losses.

3
CHILDREN AND EUTHANASIA

The best way out is always through.
—Robert Frost

Letting go of a beloved pet through euthanasia is one of the most difficult and courageous acts of kindness a pet owner will perform.

Many of us are asked to provide our pets with what is considered the final act of love and kindness, euthanasia. Although some pets do die in their sleep, most pets do not die a natural death without suffering. It is through the process of euthanasia that we can release our pets from suffering. It is through the process of grief that we ultimately free ourselves of pain and are able to fully give our hearts to another person or animal.

Living with a pet that is terminally ill or a pet that is so old it is at the end of its life can make euthanasia a consideration, which is at best a difficult experience for the entire family. Providing care for a sick pet can exhaust and drain the family of energy and financial resources, and place people on edge. However, knowing that it will soon be time to for the pet to die does allow the family time to say good-bye and help to prepare the children to do so.

Definition of Euthanasia

Children of any age need to know that euthanizing a pet is an act of courage, both loving and selfless. Most children will want a definition of euthanasia. Literally translated, euthanasia means "good death." Children should be told the pet is in the process of dying and that the veterinarian assists the pet in this process by giving the pet an injection that helps the pet to die without pain and suffering. Children should also be informed that the injection is a powerful medication that is given only by veterinarians to animals, so that the child will not fear getting a vaccination or some other type of injection.

For therapists assisting children and their parents through a loss, the following definition of euthanasia can be helpful to know. However, this definition might be too complicated for young children to understand. According to Mark Ross, D.V.M., the actual euthanasia procedure varies among veterinarians. Clients should consult their veterinarian on the way it will be performed.

The majority of small animals are given an intravenous injection of a concentrated dose of sodium pentobarbital, which produces unconsciousness within seconds. Breathing and heart function cease as a result of the profound cardiovascular depression caused by the injection of the drug. Dogs and cats are given an injection into a vein. The injection can be given directly into the abdomen or heart when a vein cannot be located. To calm an anxious pet, an oral sedative can be given prior to euthanasia.

What Should Children Be Told About Euthanasia?

A more appropriate definition of euthanasia for a very young child can be found in Marjorie Blain Parker's book *Jasper's Day*. In *Jasper's Day,* Jasper, an elderly golden retriever, has cancer and is dying. Riley, the dog's owner, is a young boy who loves Jasper and is told by his parents that he will have to say good-bye to his beloved companion. Riley and his par-

ents decide to give Jasper a special day before they take him
to be euthanized. Everything they do throughout the day
honors the life they shared together. The story, although addressing the topic of death, is a celebration of life and tenderly
addresses the issue of saying good-bye and letting go. Parker
wrote from Riley's perspective as he and his family attend
the procedure: "The veterinarian is going to give Jasper a
shot. It will be quick and gentle. For Jasper, it will be just like
going to sleep. He won't be asleep, though. Jasper will be dead.
I stand there crying. Mom, too."[1]

I often use this story to take children through the process
of saying good-bye to their pets. The story addresses Riley's
feelings of sadness and honors the bond he shared with the
dog. It describes the loss as a family loss and addresses each
person's feelings about having to euthanize Jasper. It also
teaches children that the decision to euthanize a pet is often
made out of love to release a pet from pain and suffering. In
addition, although she uses the common term for euthanasia
"put to sleep," the author addresses the fact that the dog is
not going to sleep; he will die. This is an important fact that
should be clearly stated to a child. Parker wrote from Riley's
perspective about saying good-bye: "But suddenly Jasper
whimpers. The pills must be wearing off. He's hurting. It's
time to go after all."

In *Jasper's Day,* the family is encouraged to think ahead
about the euthanasia procedure. This is important for all families that are considering euthanizing a pet. Openly discussing
how the process will go and what the children's involvement
in the process will be helps children by preparing them for
what to expect. Children who are given a role in the process,
if only hugging the dog good-bye, feel important and
significant within the family structure. Their feelings are
honored and validated. They also feel more secure knowing
that adults are in charge and are there for them and their
pet. Addressing the topic and respecting the children's feelings assists in removing some of the fear associated with
death.

Although this book focuses on helping children through pet loss, it is significant to note that children take their cue from their parents on how to cope with the issues surrounding the decision to euthanize a pet. If a parent is resolute in the decision to euthanize a terminally ill animal, a child will view it for what it is: a loving act of kindness that releases an animal from pain and suffering. However, the decision to euthanize a pet can be a complicated one. Not all parents are certain that this is the right thing to do, or when to authorize it. Often, they need more information about the process and when to perform it.

When Is the Right Time to Euthanize a Pet?

Sometimes there is only very limited time in which to authorize euthanasia for a pet that is injured and suffering. Many times this occurs when the animal is accidentally injured or taken suddenly ill and has an extremely poor prognosis for recovery. The decision to authorize euthanasia must be made on the spot and the rest of the family may not have the option to attend the procedure or to say good-bye to the pet beforehand.

Other times, the decision is one in which there is time to decide when it will take place, where it will occur, and who will attend the procedure. For some, the decision to authorize euthanasia is a given. However, other times, people may struggle with the decision and with the particulars as well. Parents who are struggling with this issue within the family setting should be encouraged to work closely with their veterinarian about when to consider euthanasia. It is important to remember that although there are requirements and indicators of when an animal should to be euthanized, there is no one, perfect, exact, right time. Families should also be referred to a pet loss support group prior to the loss. Support groups can be invaluable in assisting children and their parents when anticipating a loss and after experiencing one. In

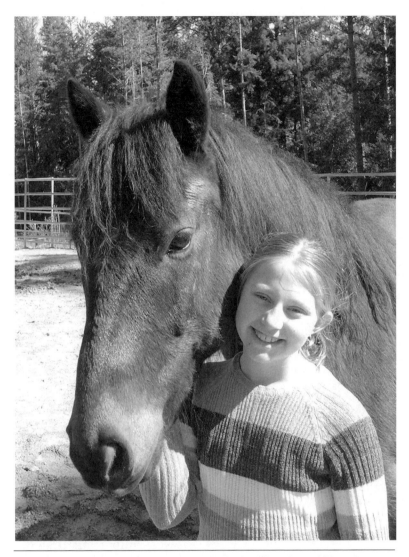

Figure 3.1 Large animal euthanasia can be extremely difficult for a child to witness.

addition, there are many books that address the topic of euthanasia, several of which are mentioned in this book. There is an extensive section on this topic in *Pet Loss and Human Emotion: Guiding Clients Through Grief* that may further inform therapists about what pet owners go through and how best to assist their clients.[2]

Preparing a Child to Say Good-bye

How the euthanasia is handled with the child can either help or hinder the process of grieving the child experiences. Children should be informed about their options in saying good-bye to their pets. Options can include having the pet euthanized at home in its favorite resting spot. A child can say good-bye to the pet at home just before it is taken to the veterinary hospital for the euthanasia procedure. A child can accompany the pet to the veterinary hospital. The child might want to have time alone with the pet in a separate room at the veterinary hospital, away from the place in which the actual procedure takes place. A child might want to view the pet's body after it is pronounced dead. Sometimes children wait to see the body until it is brought home for burial. Others might decide that they do not want to see it at all. Other children choose to attend the euthanasia procedure. Whatever the family decides, it is important to discuss available options with the veterinarian. Some veterinarians will perform at-home euthanasia, whereas others will provide the service only at their hospitals. If the procedure is to take place at the hospital, it may be wise to ask the veterinarian what time of day is better to perform the euthanasia. This way, the pet owners can have more time with the pet before and during the procedure or with the body afterward.

Many veterinarians who like working with children and their families are willing to have children present for the procedure. Others do not want children there. If the children are to attend the procedure, it is very important that the veterinarian be supportive of all family members and maintain open communication. Children should be able to ask questions and have them answered appropriately for their cognitive age by the veterinarian. Negative feelings, unanswered questions, and unfulfilled wishes can have lasting effects on the entire family. If the veterinarian is not supportive, the family may want to choose another veterinarian to perform the procedure.

Once a family talks to the veterinarian, a plan about how they will say good-bye to the pet can be made. Encourage children to discuss their wishes about how they would like to say good-bye. A discussion about burial options at this time should also be explored, depending on the child's age and level of understanding. There are as many ways to dispose of an animal's body as there are to dispose of people's bodies. Burial and cremation are common ways that pet owners release the body.

Whenever possible, children should be included in the decision-making process, if only to hear from the veterinarian that euthanasia is an option and needs to be considered for their pet. Children should also be encouraged to begin thinking about how they would like to say goodbye to the pets and way in which they would like to memorialize their cherished animals.

Large-Animal Euthanasia

Large animals are euthanized outdoors or at large-animal hospitals. An intravenous catheter is placed and the animal is given a sedative before the solution is administered. Veterinarians might attach a rope to the animal and try to lower it to the ground prior to the euthanasia. Other times the animal simply drops. This can be disturbing for a child to see. Again, in deciding whether a child should attend the euthanasia procedure of a large animal, all the same considerations for small-animal euthanasia apply.

How a Support Group Can Help Families to Prepare

In a pet loss support group, families can gain valuable knowledge about the grieving process and how to assist children through a loss. Families are able to meet other pet owners who are anticipating a loss or who have recently experienced a pet loss. The fact that a pet loss support group exists helps to validate the significance of this type of loss and offers a forum in which pet owners can explore their feelings and receive emotional support.

The following is a case example that illustrates how a support group can assist a family when a loss is anticipated.

The Jones Family: Peggy, Greg, Annabelle, Austin, and Arliss

Arliss was a 2-year-old cat with feline leukemia. He had survived two illnesses in the past 6 months. When he became ill for a third time, Arliss's veterinarian prescribed another round of antibiotics to treat the infection and suggested the family consider euthanasia for him. The family attended a pet loss support group to address the issue of euthanasia and to come to an agreement about when and if it should be performed.

Peggy and Greg, 11-year-old Annabelle's and 15-year-old Austin's parents, discussed the family's love for Arliss. They spoke affectionately to the group about the cat and how they had first gotten him. The family also spoke of the their other two cats at home. One of the cats, Tyson, was a particular favorite of Austin. The other cat, Marigold, was liked and loved but was more aloof and spent a great deal of time on her own. Arliss was an indoor cat who spent the majority of his time with the family. The parents told of their surprise when they discovered that Arliss had feline leukemia. They said that he tested negative as a young kitten and had been vaccinated against the disease. The other two cats at home had also been tested and vaccinated, and were tested negative a second time.

Although Arliss was responding favorably to the current round of medication, the family was cautioned that he would most likely become ill again in the near future and might not survive. The therapist asked each person in the family if he or she would want to euthanize Arliss if he were suffering and would not recover. Each person said yes.

Annabelle pointed out that Arliss was getting better. When the therapist acknowledged that Annabelle and the rest of the family felt hopeful because Arliss was doing better,

Annabelle chimed in with all the things that she and Arliss would do together in the near future. Austin reminded her that Arliss might not live much longer. The therapist acknowledged this fact. Annabelle began to cry, and the therapist commented that she saw the tears on Annabelle's cheeks. Annabelle replied defensively, "Yeah, so?" Annabelle picked up her chair and completely turned it toward her father so that her back was to the therapist when she sat down. She swung her legs and fidgeted in her chair. She clearly demonstrated her anger at having to face the possible loss of her beloved cat. Her response and behavior poignantly demonstrated her need to focus on the fact that Arliss was getting better and her hope that he would live a long time. The therapist used this time to discuss another stage of grieving, which is anger.

Greg inquired as to the other stages of grief and the order in which they could expect to go through them. The therapist told him that whereas Elisabeth Kubler-Ross had written about the stages and other therapists had also written about stages, the process of grief was not linear and they might not be experienced in order. Some stages might not be experienced at all. However, denial is one of the first stages and acceptance or resolution is one of the final stages. Greg asked if the loss of their pet was something they would eventually "get over." The therapist said that she thought it was not something they would necessarily get over, but it was something they would get through. They would always remember the loss and the life they shared with Arliss, but at some point the pain would lessen and they would be able to remember Arliss with joy. She commented again on the importance of coming together as a family and respecting each person's way of grieving and demonstrating feelings. People grieve at different rates. Some people get through it much sooner than others.

The therapist asked Austin if there were any issues about loss they had not addressed in the group. Austin said yes. He was very concerned about his cat Tyson getting leukemia. The therapist asked the parents if they had asked the veterinarian about the other cats getting the virus. They said yes and told Austin that the veterinarian felt that because Tyson had been vaccinated and exposed and had recently tested negative, he most likely would not get the virus. Austin showed relief at this news.

The therapist explained that when one pet we love becomes ill, it is normal to be concerned about the health and well-being of other pets too. This could be applied to people as well, but because the children did not bring up concern about their health or their parents' health, she decided not to address this point.

Annabelle asked to hear from the man who was sitting in a chair near her. She said that he had not had a turn to talk about his loss. The man, Bill, was at first uncomfortable as he shared his regret at not euthanizing his dog. He said that he felt that because of his failure to authorize the euthanasia and what he deemed selfishness at hanging on too long, his dog suffered. Austin listened intently. Austin said that he would not allow that to happen to Arliss.

The group discussed one of the stages of grief, denial, and how it was important to help cushion the impact of learning that your pet has a terminal disease but how it also could make it difficult to know when to authorize euthanasia. Bill said that while facing the loss of his current dog, he had appointed an advocate, a friend, who would tell him when he thought the dog was suffering. Bill said that he felt that this would help him to avoid making the same mistake that he made with his first dog. Bill said before his first dog died, his veterinarian had told him that he would know when it was time to bring the dog in to be euthanized. Bill explained though that when he was caring for this sick pet he had focused only on the positive and refused to see the negative— the dog's suffering. As a result, he waited too long to relieve that suffering. The therapist acknowledged that when one is caught up in trying to care for a sick pet, it is easy to lose sight of the big picture and to see the overall quality of the pet's life. Appointing a close friend to be the dog's advocate (a person who sees the dog through different eyes) or checking in frequently with the veterinarian are ways to avoid letting the pet suffer.

Greg said he thought that of the four of them, Peggy would handle the loss best. When asked why, he said it was because she had already gone through the loss of her mother, brother, father, and childhood dog, whereas this was the first loss for him, Annabelle, and Austin. Peggy said that she thought she would grieve for Arliss as much as they would, if not more, because she was so attached to him. The therapist acknowledged that although Peggy did have more experience with loss, going through another loss was like peeling back the layers of an onion. Each loss echoes a previous loss and comes with its own experiences, memories, and possible unresolved feelings.

The therapist acknowledged Peggy's previous losses and validated them by explaining that although a person can draw on what worked and did not work in getting through an earlier loss, new losses can bring up past feelings that can complicate working through the current loss. However, a new loss can also be an opportunity to bring closure to past losses. Peggy was asked to share what she had learned from her past losses. She said that although they were the most intensely felt painful experiences of her life, the feelings eventually did subside and she had been able to move on. The therapist discussed the fact that although the pain initially feels like something a person might never get through, eventually he or she does and is able to remember the life shared with the pet or person and to feel joy at having done so.

Peggy discussed the loss of her father and her dog. When she talked about her dog Apples, who had drowned in her father's swimming pool shortly before her father died, Annabelle walked over to her with tissues in hand and asked her if she was going to cry about Apples. Peggy told her that she was not going to cry and that she had worked through the loss long ago, but she did regret the way he died. Annabelle learned that her mother was able to remember, without tears, the life she shared with Apples.

The therapist used this point in the session as an opportunity to commend the family on their coming together to work through their feelings about learning that Arliss had a terminal illness. The therapist also explained to the parents the importance of laying a solid foundation of coping skills that their children could use for future losses.

She talked about how death is not the only type of loss people experience. Losing a job, moving, going to another school, or losing a friendship are all losses. Annabelle told Austin that he had experienced a recent loss, but Austin was not sure what she was talking about. Annabelle told him that when his friend Kevin moved to England, that was a loss. Austin said that they were still friends, and Annabelle reminded him that they were not able to see each other and that Austin missed him. Austin said that was true, and Peggy, realizing how much Austin missed the friendship, suggested that he call Kevin on the phone. They discussed the fact that a friend moving to another country was indeed a loss even though it differed from loss involving death.

The family discussed ways in which they could keep Arliss's memory alive. They decided that they wanted to take more pictures of him and place them in a scrapbook. Peggy and Annabelle shared the hobby of making scrapbooks. Annabelle said that she wanted to include photos of other animals too. Her parents agreed. The therapist suggested that they might want to write down some of the memories they had about Arliss. She recommended a book titled *My Personal Pet Remembrance Journal,* by Enid Samuel Traisman.[3]

Toward the end of the group session, Annabelle, clearly done with the session, said it was time to leave. She got up and pushed her chair toward a table and then walked around the room as the family said their good-byes. The therapist took into consideration her need to end the discussion for now and move on to other things. The family said that they would attend the group the following week to discuss the parameters for deciding when to euthanize Arliss and to work through more of their feelings.

The following week the family inquired about the actual euthanasia procedure. Regarding having the children attend the euthanasia procedure, Greg said that he did not feel it was appropriate. Austin chimed in and said that he wanted to be there with Arliss to comfort him during the process. The therapist asked the parents if the veterinarian had explained the process. They said no. The therapist then asked them if she could explain the process, and they agreed. The therapist described the actual procedure. She also told about the possibility that the process might not go as planned. Although this occurs only a small percentage of the time, it is important to prepare people for what they might witness. She described the method as quick and painless, similar to what it looks like when someone falls asleep, but said that the pet's internal organs quickly shut down and they die. She made the distinction between sleeping and dying. She also said that sometimes the veterinarian might experience difficulty finding a vein (when a catheter is not used) and he or she might have to place a catheter in the pet. The therapist also let the family know that although they may choose to attend or not to attend, people often changed their minds when faced with the moment. It was perfectly fine to choose to leave or to ask to attend at that moment.

She also said that a parent might need to attend to a child and leave the pet or support a child through the procedure. Often times it is a good idea to as a close family friend to go with the family to assist the children if the parents are overcome with their emotions or are unwilling to leave the pet during the procedure—as is often the process when children attend the birth of a sibling. The therapist encouraged the family to discuss their concerns and their wishes with the veterinarian prior to the euthanasia procedure.

The process of grieving usually begins when the child is told that the pet is terminal. The dying process may be short or long. Keeping a pet comfortable that is very ill can be an exhausting and stressful experience. Parents may become short tempered, have less time for their children, feel anxious about the pet's quality of life, and wonder if they are properly caring for the pet. They might become very tired from interrupted sleep. The entire family will feel the stress of the effort that is required to care for a sick animal. As a result, it is not uncommon for children who have gone through this, and in essence kept a deathwatch over a pet, to feel a sense of relief when the pet dies. They might say, "I'm glad he's gone." This does not mean that they did not love the pet. They are expressing relief at not having to live with the burden of caring for a sick or elderly pet. This honest expression should not be discouraged. It should not be assumed that children who express their relief from the tension that preceded the death do not feel sadness over the pet's death.

Children also might feel angry at a sick or elderly pet. They may think that the pet is choosing to die or to leave them. Open communication between the child and the parents or therapist should encourage any questions about this and allow the child to fully understand what it is that is happening during the death process. A caregiver might want to say to a child who is refusing to say good-bye to a pet that is dying (especially if the child is angry at the pet for "abandoning" him or her) something like, "I know that you love Rigby and Rigby knows that you love him. You've been a wonderful a pet owner and have taken very good care of him." The caregiver might offer to let the child write the pet a note and say good-bye without seeing the pet.

Should a Child Attend the Euthanasia Procedure?

Of all of the issues surrounding death and dying and children, whether children should attend the euthanasia of a beloved pet is one of the most hotly debated. There are compelling reasons supporting both sides of this issue. Some professionals say that attending a euthanasia procedure can have adverse emotional effects on children. Others argue that permitting children to experience and express grief in a supportive setting can establish a healthy foundation on which to build for future losses.

Children should be included in the decision-making process regarding euthanasia for their pet, whether or not they attend the euthanasia procedure. Taking them out of the decision-making process in an attempt to spare them the guilt of having to decide on euthanasia for their pet only serves to reinforce their feelings of guilt about not being able to help their pet by ending its suffering.

When addressing this issue, a caregiver must take into consideration the child's past experiences with loss, family dynamics, cognitive level of understanding and awareness, and support systems. The caregivers' and veterinarian's willingness and ability to support the child through a procedure must also be taken into consideration. A veterinarian who is not comfortable having a child witness the procedure might not be able to answer questions about the medical procedure or help to create a safe environment in which the child feels nurtured and protected at a time when he or she might be feeling most vulnerable. This is also true of parents or other caregivers. If they are not comfortable in having their child witness and take part in the final stages of the pet's life, then the child will not have the support he or she needs to participate in death experiences. Like children who are allowed to witness the birth of a sibling, a child who attends a euthanasia procedure must also be prepared for what he or she will see. Like birth, the death process can be filled with unanticipated happenings. Children and their caregivers should be educated about what to expect and what their role will be in assisting with the euthanasia.

Children mature enough to assist with the care of a sick or elderly pet should be allowed to be involved in the euthanasia decision and in deciding whether to attend the procedure. However, children should be provided with a detailed description of the procedure, how it happens, what happens to the pet's body, and when and where the procedure will take place. Once a child is given this information, his or her decision whether to participate should be respected. Sometimes children will change their mind right before the procedure is to begin, either choosing not to attend or deciding to attend. Parents should be prepared for this change of events and be able to support their child either way. It is often a good idea to bring another adult to the procedure, someone who can be there for the child, either to remove the child from the procedure and stay with him or her or to bring the child into the procedure and support him or her emotionally while it is happening.

With both large- and small-animal euthanasia there is always the chance, although infrequent, that the procedure will not go smoothly. In the absence of an intravenous catheter (which is usually administered to the animal in a separate room outside of where the euthanasia takes place), it might take several attempts to find a vein. There can be agonal breathing, loss of bladder control, reflexive muscle contractions, and vocalization. Parents and their children who might want to attend should be prepared for these possibilities before making a final decision about being present for the euthanasia procedure.

Parents and children who do not want to see the actual procedure might want to come in to see the pet's body and to say their final good-byes after the procedure has been performed. Veterinarians and their staff are often sensitive to the needs of pet owners and are willing to accommodate their needs as they work through their grief.

The following example demonstrates how two children and their parents witnessed the euthanasia of their dog.

Tim, Joyce, Brandon, Katie, and Peanut

Tim and Joyce had two children—Brandon, age 8, and Katie, age 6—and a 17-year-old dog named Peanut. Peanut had been a member of the family since he was a puppy, and the family shared a common love for him. The dog was dying of complications related to old age. He could no longer stand and he had problems with bladder control. Tim and Joyce had talked with the children ahead of time and, along with the veterinarian, compassionately explained what the euthanasia procedure would involve.

Brandon and Katie were given the choice of attending the euthanasia procedure, saying good-bye to Peanut beforehand, or coming into the room after the procedure to say their final good-byes. Both children chose to be present during the procedure.

The entire family went to the veterinary clinic with Peanut. The veterinarian told the family he thought they were doing the best thing for Peanut by allowing him to have a peaceful death. He then asked the family if they were ready for him to give Peanut the injection. They all nodded yes.

The family gently stroked Peanut while the veterinarian administered the injection. Peanut slowly wagged his tail against the table. In a matter of seconds, Peanut's body became still. The veterinarian listened to Peanut's heart. Everyone in the room was silent. When the veterinarian said that Peanut was dead, Katie began to cry. Joyce held her close as she wept. Brandon was silent and looked from one person to another in disbelief. Tim told Brandon that Peanut was gone now and that he was relieved of the pain he had felt. Brandon pressed his face against his mother's skirt and silently sobbed. Tim's eyes filled with tears. The children slowly moved from their mom and went to pet Peanut's lifeless body.

Brandon spent a lot of time staring into Peanut's open eyes. He asked, "If he's dead, how come his eyes are open? Can he

see us?" The veterinarian explained that animals usually died
with their eyes open, and that Peanut could not see or hear
them anymore. Tim and Joyce chose this time to explain
their spiritual beliefs to the children regarding death. They
told Brandon and Katie that Peanut's spirit had been set free—
that the part that had housed his spirit was his body, and
that was all that was left of him here. Joyce told the children
they could keep Peanut's memory alive by remembering all
the times they had shared with Peanut. Joyce and Tim then
shared a story about when they adopted Peanut as a puppy.

Drawing from a children's story called *The Tenth Good
Thing About Barney,* by Judith Viorst, Joyce and Tim asked
the children to remember 10 good things about Peanut.[4] Brandon said that Peanut was a good friend. He urged his mom to
tell some good things. Joyce said Peanut never bit anyone.
She recalled how he loved to run in an open field near their
house. Katie said he was nice, and Tim agreed.

The family was ready to leave, when Brandon suddenly
asked if they had done the right thing for Peanut in authorizing the euthanasia. Tim and Joyce were surprised by the question. Both parents and the veterinarian reassured Brandon
that it was not only the right thing to do but also a loving and
unselfish act. Katie gave Peanut one last hug good-bye, and
the family left.

Two weeks later, Tim and Joyce reported that the children
had accepted Peanut's death and did not seem to be experiencing any adverse effects from having been present at the
procedure. This can be attributed to the parents' having made
the children aware of Peanut's deteriorating condition before
he was euthanzied. This is very important in preparing children for the loss of a pet.

The children were included in the process by participating in the decision for euthanasia, being allowed to voice their
concerns and fears, and being given options about how they
could say good-bye to Peanut. The veterinarian was also supportive and helpful. Most significant was the support, open-

ness, and honesty Tim and Joyce gave to their children. They took time to encourage Brandon and Katie to ask questions and to share their grief, and they provided them with information in terms they could understand.[5]

Convenience and Behavioral Problem Euthanasia

The term *convenience euthanasia* is misleading. It implies that the pet owner wants to terminate the life of a pet simply because he or she no longer wants to take responsibility for it. In some extreme cases this is true. However, most veterinarians will not administer euthanasia to a healthy pet unless there are other factors involved. Pet owners can choose euthanasia for a variety of reasons. One of the reasons to euthanize that might be the most difficult to help a child understand is when a pet has become destructive and is a danger to others.

Although unusual, there are cases when a family pet develops a severe behavior problem. Sometimes the problem can be corrected through a combination of medication and behavior modification training. Other times, pet owners find that they have exhausted all possible means of getting the animal to change its behavior. When the behavior is harmful to people (e.g., biting) or to other animals (e.g., attacking another family pet) or is destructive (e.g., inappropriately marking territory, urinating on the carpet and furniture, chewing the walls or furniture), other options must be considered. One of these options is to euthanize the pet. Families considering this option need particular support. They need to know that they have done everything in their power to help the animal. They might feel guilty about authorizing the procedure and be torn between their love for their pet and their responsibility to other family members. Children who have witnessed the animal's behavior and even fear the pet can still have a difficult time understanding why the pet has to be euthanized.

Young children might fear that if their pet can be euthanized because of behavior problems, then something bad could happen to them if they are not well behaved. Children need to be told that although we consider our pets to be family members, they are not humans. As animals, they respond differently and behave differently from people. Although very young children might bite, scratch, or do other hurtful things, as humans they can be taught to behave differently. Some animals might not be able to learn new behaviors and stop biting, destroying property, or marking their territory inappropriately (e.g., urinating on the furniture or carpet).

Connor and Candy

Connor was a very good boy, too well behaved, after his dog, a 3-year-old mixed breed named Candy, was euthanized for attacking a child who lived on their street. Connor, age 8, and his parents had adopted Candy from some neighbors who moved a year earlier. Candy had adapted to her new family. She and Connor became friends and would spend time every day after school playing ball. Soon after adopting her, it became apparent to the family that Candy was very protective of them. When they took her for walks, Candy would often growl at children and adults who approached the family. A couple of times Candy snapped at a child who tried to pet her. The parents sought help from their veterinarian and were referred to an animal behaviorist. Together they worked with the behaviorist and the veterinarian to extinguish the aggressive behavior.

Attempts to change Candy's aggressive behavior toward nonfamily members failed. Candy was confined to the backyard. Connor's parents were concerned that Candy might hurt Connor if the right set of circumstances came into play. They allowed Connor to play with the dog only under their supervision.

One afternoon Candy got out of the yard through an open gate. Connor and his mother saw her leave and gave chase.

They caught Candy. Just as they were attaching her to a leash, a young girl approached them and tried to pet Candy before the mother could tell her not to do so. Candy bit the girl on the face. Horrified, the mother and father decided that they no longer wanted to take responsibility for Candy. They contacted their veterinarian and decided to euthanize the dog. Connor was told of the decision and told that he would get another dog soon. He was also allowed to say good-bye to Candy just before his father took him to the veterinarian's office.

At first Connor seemed to be fine. He showed no outward signs of grief. He attended school and talked about the new dog—"the one that wouldn't bite anyone, *ever*"—that he was going to get. In fact, recalling his good-bye to Candy, his mother said that he seemed angry with Candy rather than sad that he was losing her. He talked about how his dog was "bad" and bad dogs could not live with them.

Connor's mother contacted a therapist when Connor's behavior changed so dramatically at home that he was no longer the easygoing boy who sometimes got into trouble. The new Connor was overly concerned about doing everything perfectly, and he constantly asked his parents if he was being "good."

After his third play therapy session, Connor showed the therapist what happened to bad dogs that bite. He chose a stuffed dog and made it bite a doll. He punished the dog by shooting it with a toy gun. He said, "Now you're dead!" Connor revealed in the session his deepest fear, that if he was not well behaved, his parents might get rid of him too.

The therapist continued to work with Connor by educating him about what euthanasia was. Sometimes children and adults imagine that it is far worse than a lethal injection administered by a veterinarian. The therapist also worked with the family to reassure Connor. They helped him to understand how animals and people are different, and they explained that a dog that is aggressive and attacks other people sometimes cannot be helped. They also let Connor know the many ways in which they tried to help Candy stop biting and why they felt that if they gave her to another home, she might continue to severely hurt other people. They let Connor know that even though they loved and cared about Candy, Connor was their first priority. They also told him that although they felt that they did the right thing in euthanizing Candy, they did miss the wonderful things they loved about her. They shared their grief with Connor and in turn allowed Connor to express his grief over his loss.

Conclusion

Most of the time when euthanasia is advised, the family has time to say good-bye to the pet. Preparing children for the loss is paramount in assisting them through the grieving process. There are times when well-intentioned parents might avoid the issue of euthanasia with their children in an attempt to protect them. However, telling the child the pet died in its sleep, ran away, or was given to a farmer who loves dogs or some other story meant to help children not have to face the truth about a loss is worse than telling the truth. Children learn to distrust adults when adults lie to them. They also hear more and know more than we give them credit for. They need to be helped and shown how to face a loss and work through it.

It is important to create an environment of open communication, one in which the child feels safe to ask questions about the impending loss. Lies, avoidance, and trivializing the loss only serve to create problems for the child and impede the process of grieving.

For the majority of pet owners, there is never a perfect or right time for an animal to be euthanized. The decision to euthanize a pet should be seen on a continuum. Many pet owners are concerned with making the decision too soon or waiting too long. Pet owners should be encouraged to work closely with their veterinarians regarding the decision to euthanize a pet. In addition, children should be included in the decision-making process, if only to be made aware of the fact that this will happen. Terms such as *put down* or *put to sleep* should be avoided. Children should be told that the pet will be put to death and that euthanasia is a loving and unselfish act that helps the pet to die with dignity and without enduring needless suffering.

Children will grow into adults who have to face many types of losses throughout their lives. If they become pet owners, euthanasia will probably be one of the types of losses they have to face. Adults who were sheltered from the death process as children will have difficulty working through a loss. Although it is true that euthanasia is a complicated topic that is difficult to explain to children, it is a part of the process of death that children need help in understanding. It should not be viewed as something that is shameful or wrong. Euthanasia is a final act of love, one that takes courage to authorize by people who care for animals, regardless if it is performed to release an ill pet from suffering or to release a pet who has extreme behavior problems that place people and other animals at risk for injury or death.

4
SPECIAL TYPES OF LOSS

The basic fact is that humanity survives through kindness, love and compassion. That human beings can develop these qualities is their real blessing.

—The Dalai Lama

Teaching children about loss and working through all the manifestations of grief not only assists children in becoming mature adults who possess healthy coping skills, it also teaches them about kindness, love, and compassion toward animals, themselves, and other human beings.

Special types of loss often involve feelings of anger and guilt, and it can be more difficult to assist a child through the process of grieving such losses. Special losses can also offer the opportunity to teach a child about compassion toward others, and especially toward oneself. The ability to feel is an integral part of being human. Children are born with the ability to feel. They take their cues about how to direct and interpret those feelings from the adults who care for them. Sometimes parents avoid the topic of pet loss with a child because they cannot bear to face the intensity of their child's emotions. This can be especially true when the loss involves special circumstances (gruesome details, or involvement in the death on the part of the child or other family members). As a result, the child's unwillingness to accept the loss and to grieve it is reinforced by the protective attitude of the parent(s).

Although the majority of pet losses occur because the animal is euthanized, there are many ways in which a pet loss can occur. A child might need long-term support when the loss is unresolved, as when a pet goes missing. The way in which a pet dies can bring up particular questions, fears, and anxieties for a child. Giving a pet to a new home is another instance in which children need to express their feelings and grief over the loss. The child might even feel responsible for the loss if the pet is to be given away because the child is allergic to the animal. Often a pet loss is the by-product of a parental divorce, when parents may need to move from a house into a rental property where animals are not allowed. Sometimes pets are accidentally injured or killed by children. These are some of the special types of loss that we explore in this section.

Divorce

When divorce happens, families are often faced with numerous changes. Some of these changes can affect the family's ability to care for a pet. Families may need to move into a new place that does not allow pets, or the parents might have a significant reduction in income that does not allow them to adequately provide for a pet. Any of these factors can result in having to find a new home for the pet. In addition, children going through a divorce are experiencing numerous changes and many losses all at once. They are losing the family structure that they have always known. They may have to move, change schools, or adjust to living with a stepparent and stepsiblings. Losing a beloved companion animal that has been a friend and confidant over the years only compounds this loss, putting children at risk for depression, anxiety, and behavior problems. Ideally, if at all possible, children should be allowed to keep their pets during such periods. If this is not possible, caregivers should assist children in expressing all of their feelings, including anger, and allow them to say good-bye to their pets.

Children who are experiencing multiple losses can be tired, cranky, angry, and moody. They might fight with siblings and have difficulty sleeping and eat too much or too little. They can seem too well behaved, wanting to take care of parents and other siblings. It is important that consistent routines, friends, and extended family members remain in a child's life. Children will find comfort in maintaining the same bedtime routine, participating in extracurricular activities that have brought them pleasure, and spending time with family and friends with whom they share a positive relationship. If a child has difficulty eating or sleeping for more than a couple of weeks, the child should be assessed for depression by a physician or child psychiatrist (please see chapter 8 on therapeutic interventions).

There are times when a pet's death coincides with a divorce. The death of the pet, although significant in itself, can also become a representation of the death of the family structure. Even though a new structure will be born from the divorce, it is important to realize that children will grieve everything at once and this grief will be intensely felt. Children might feel as if "everything has died." Although an intense display of emotion can seem overly dramatic to parents, children should be encouraged to fully express themselves and let their feelings out over a period of time. Children might feel angry with their parents, angry with God, or angry at life and might become angry at the pet for dying and leaving them. Encourage children to work through their feelings by gently commenting on them. For example, if the child said that he does not care that Murphy is dead because he hated him, a caregiver might say, "I hear you saying that you are really angry with Murphy." Do not try to talk the child out of his feelings. Let him express to you what he is feeling and help him to work through the pain by acknowledging and validating his feelings.

Children who do experience the loss of a pet during this time (through the pet's dying, being adopted, or running away) should be provided with the support necessary to work through all of their losses. Often, even with the most supportive and loving parents, a child's feelings can be overlooked when parents are going through the strains of ending a relationship and beginning new lives. Providing a child with additional means of support is often best, especially when the child must adjust to the loss of a pet as well.

Teachers, school counselors, pediatricians, and caregivers should be notified and made aware of all of the changes in the child's life and asked to respect the child's feelings and to be understanding. Children who are experiencing compound losses can have difficulty concentrating, short attention spans, and trouble socializing. They might withdraw socially, perform poorly on schoolwork, and regress emotionally.

Children who are supported and provided with appropriate interventions as needed through the death or loss of a pet and the experience of their parents' divorce can successfully work through the losses and can turn their attention to their new lives and new experiences that will come.

When a Child Accidentally Harms or Kills a Pet

Accidents are an unfortunate part of life. Because they take us by surprise, they leave us feeling vulnerable and confused. Often we can learn from accidents through hindsight and prevent future ones. Pets have been the unfortunate victims of accidents involving cars, garage doors, pools, tangled leashes, cage doors being left ajar, being left out in the sun too long, and being stepped on. Children who unintentionally harm their pets are also victims. They are old enough to understand that their actions caused the demise of their pets but are too young to know how to forgive themselves and to cope with complicated grief.

The following case example illustrates the complex feelings children face when having accidentally harmed their pets.

Erica and Mickey

Erica, a 14-year-old girl, had adopted Mickey, her 2-year-old dachshund, when he was just 6 months old. Erica was homeschooled by her mother and had lots of time to spend with Mickey. Erica and her mother often took Mickey to her father's office to visit. Erica referred to Mickey as her best friend and said he was "like a child." Erica's mother said that they had also had a dog when Erica was 6 years old who died from a heart attack. Erica said that the dog died while playing Frisbee in the yard with her. The family had waited to get another dog until Erica was old enough to take more responsibility for the pet. When Erica was 13, she adopted Mickey and made a promise to Mickey and to her parents that she would be responsible for him and take very good care of him.

She said that because Mickey was small she was very concerned about his well-being. She once refused to take Mickey to her cousin's house because she was afraid the younger children there might accidentally harm Mickey. She often carried Mickey in her purse or walked him on a leash attached to his harness. One afternoon, she and her mother were getting ready to take Mickey for a walk. She attached his leash to his harness, when the doorbell rang. Excitedly, Mickey jumped up and down and ran around Erica's feet. The leash became tangled around Erica's legs as Mickey bounced and barked at the caller at the door. Erica attempted to untangle the leash, started to fall, and accidentally stepped on Mickey. Her mother watched in horror as Erica tried desperately to contort her body to avoid futher injuring Mickey. Erica fell into a nearby table, hurting her leg, and falling on Mickey. Mickey lay unconscious on the floor.

Erica and her mother rushed Mickey to the veterinary hospital. Mickey was comatose. The emergency veterinarian told Erica and her mother that there was little hope and that they should consider euthanizing Mickey. After consulting with Mickey's regular veterinarian, the family decided to give Mickey a few more days to see if he might come out of the

coma. Erica and her mother attended the pet loss support
group to prepare for the possible loss of Mickey and to work
through the guilt Erica said that she felt over Mickey's condition. Erica's father chose not to attend. Erica said that her
father found it difficult to talk about the accident with her,
although he had purchased a small dachshund statue for her
and left it for her to find in the morning. Erica's mother said
that this was her husband's way of demonstrating that he
cared. Erica said that although she was touched by the gift,
she wished that she could talk to her father about what had
happened to Mickey. She said that she blamed herself for not
being more careful.

Erica's mother said that Erica was experiencing difficulty
eating and sleeping and was not able to concentrate on her
schoolwork. She was concerned about her daughter's well-
being and saddened about Mickey's condition. The therapist
acknowledged that they had come to the support group hopeful
that Mickey might come out of the coma (Mickey's veterinarian had given him a 50-50 chance) and to work through the
guilt that Erica felt over the accident. The mother also acknowledged that they might be preparing for Mickey's death.

At this point Erica began to cry. She told the group how
much she loved Mickey and wished that she could go back to
that moment when he was injured and change the outcome.
She said that she blamed herself for not being more careful.
She recounted Mickey's accident in detail. The therapist
pointed out that Erica had been taking precautions with
Mickey by putting his leash on when taking him for a walk.
She also reminded Erica that she had decided to not take
Mickey over to her cousin's house because of concerns for
his safety there. She reminded Erica of the facts that her
mother shared with the group about how carefully Erica took
care of Mickey. An adult in the group gently pointed out to
Erica that an accident is something that is not planned and
is not wanted or unintended; it is an unfortunate happening
despite the best of intentions.

Erica shared with the group that she thought she had killed her first dog. Her mother was surprised by this admission. Erica said that if she had not been playing Frisbee with her dog, he might not have had a heart attack. Erica's mother was able to explain to her that although Erica had not ben told, because she was very young at the time, the dog had an underlying heart condition since birth and could have died at any time. The fact that Erika had been playing with him at the time of his death made no difference. Erica showed in her posture a sense of relief at having learned this.

Erica shared with the group how difficult it was to see Mickey lying in the hospital in a coma. She had told Mickey how sorry she was and how she loved him. She was not sure if he could hear her, though. The therapist commented on how much Erica cared for Mickey and how much Mickey must care for her. Erica said that she thought Mickey cared for her a lot. The therapist then asked Erica if she thought Mickey would want her to blame herself. Erica thought about it and said, "No." The therapist asked her if she could choose to let go of her guilt and continue to give her love to Mickey. She said she would try.

Erica's mother told Erica that it was difficult to see her in so much pain. She told her that she loved her and in no way blamed her for what had happened to either dog. Then Erica's mother asked if she could pray with her for Mickey to get well. Erica said that she had try praying but she was not sure she believed it would help Mickey. She thought that she could sit with Mickey in the hospital, pet him, and tell him how much she wanted him to get well.

The therapist acknowledged that although Mickey might not die, there was also a chance that he might not fully re-cover. She asked Erica and her mother if they and their vet-erinarian had established some boundaries regarding euthanasia. Erica's mother said that they, along with their veterinarian, were going to wait over the weekend to see if there was any improvement in Mickey's condition. Erica and her mother said that if Mickey did not show signs of improvement, they would return to the group the following week.

One week after the group meeting, the therapist learned that Mickey had come out of his coma and would be able to return home. Although Erica did not experience the loss of this pet, she was able to work through the feelings of guilt she had regarding her role in the accident and some of the unresolved feelings she possessed from the loss of her first dog. She had blamed herself for his death because she was playing with him at the time that he died. Now more mature and able to understand more, she was able to use the experience with Mickey to ask her mother more questions about the loss of her first dog and learn that she was in no way responsible for it. She also was able to forgive herself for the role she had played in Mickey's accident.

When a child has a role in a pet's demise, it is vital that the caregivers carefully consider how they respond and what they say to the child regarding the accident or loss. Children should be encouraged to openly discuss what happened and how they feel about it. They might hide certain facts or interpret them incorrectly because they want to disguise their guilt or because they fear a negative repercussion. In Erica's case, she had carried the burden of guilt over the death of her first dog with her for many years. Had she been able to share her feelings regarding her role in the death of her first dog, then she might have been able to work through the guilt soon after she experienced the loss.

Accidental Loss of a Pet

Children can internalize feelings of inadequacy and self-blame over what parents and other adults may deem as trivial events involving a pet loss. For example, a young child who was cleaning out her fish bowl accidentally placed the fish in water that was too warm and they died. The mother's response to her—"I told you to be careful"—caused her to blame herself and feel guilty over the loss of her pet fish. It was not until she was an adult, working through the loss of another pet in the pet loss support group, that she was able finally to acknowledge and work through her feelings over the loss of her fish. Often, adults who care for children may not stop to consider their responses and how children can interpret them, especially if the adult spoke out of frustration or anger.

Adult caregivers must also consider their own roles in the demise of pets. Children who are young have limited abilities in caring for pets. It is not realistic to expect even elementary-school-age children to accept sole responsibility in caring for a pet. It is normal for young children to forget to walk, feed, clean up after, and contain their pets. Parents must accept full responsibility for the care and well-being of any animal that they allow their child to have for a pet. It is the responsibility of the caregiver to teach the skills necessary to help children learn to take care of the animals they love and to supervise this care as the children mature.

The following example illustrates one child's protective feelings toward a new pet after the tragic loss of another pet.

Trevor and Rory

Trevor was 8 years old when his 12-week-old kitten Rory was hit by a car and died on Christmas Eve. Trevor's parents were out buying a Christmas tree and Trevor and Rory were at home being cared for by a babysitter. When the babysitter opened the front door the kitten ran outside and into the street. The kitten was run over by a car. Trevor was inside playing and did not see the accident. A next-door neighbor saw it happen and cleaned up Rory's remains. He took the pet's body to his home. When the parents arrived, the babysitter told them what had happened. She also told them that she had not told Trevor.

Trevor was very upset by the news and wanted to see Rory's body. However, the neighbor cautioned them against opening the bag, as the accident had severely damaged Rory's body. The parents explained to Trevor that they would not want him to remember Rory's body in the condition it was in and they were certain that they did not want Trevor to see it. They did show Trevor the bag. The three of them decided to send Rory's remains to be cremated. A couple of weeks after receiving the ashes, they buried Rory's ashes in their backyard.

When Trevor was 12 years old he asked his parents for another kitten. Soon after, someone left a box of kittens at his father's veterinary office. His father chose a tenacious kitten with a cute personality. He presented the kitten to his son. His son named him Murray. Murray and Trevor were constant companions. When the kitten was a year old the father suggested to Trevor that they allow Murray to play outside in the backyard, because the cat often cried at the door when Trevor went out.

Trevor became very upset and said, "No." When his parents questioned him about his decision to keep Murray inside the house, he told them that he was afraid Murray would be killed.

Although the parents realized that Murray would be safer inside, and that they would support Trevor's decision to remain him as an indoor cat, they also decided to address Trevor's concerns and work through any feelings he might still have over the loss of Rory. After a period of time, Murray did escape to the backyard through an open door a few times, and Trevor's mom reported that Trevor did not seem overly concerned when returning Murray to the house.

Missing Pets

When pets are lost or stolen, children are left to wonder what the fate of their pet might be. In many cases the fate of the pet is never discovered. Caregivers should assist children in their effort to find the pet. Posting flyers providing information about the pet, visiting local animal shelters to look for the pet, and asking neighbors if they have seen the pet will assist children by empowering them to help find the pet. Pets are found and do get returned to their owners. Sometimes pets turn up several weeks or even months later. However, many other times the pet is gone and the fate of the pet remains unknown. Children may attempt to cling to the hope of the pet's return, they may become angry at the pet for leaving them, and they may wonder what role they played, if any, in the loss of the pet. They can even become fearful that they too can be taken from their home. Children might decide to create a story about what might have happened to the pet.

Creating a story allows the child to find closure in the loss. However, an adult should not make up a story about the pet's fate and tell the child that is what happened. As children mature, and their intellectual capacity increases, they can easily see through the lie and view it as a betrayal on their parent's part instead of a gesture of goodwill made to help the child achieve closure. Also, although it is the job of the therapist to help the client invent an ending to the story with which he or she can live with, it is important to note that the child should be allowed and encouraged to work through his or her feelings and arrive at his or her own conclusions. Whatever the conclusion the child chooses, adults should support the child through the grieving process in arriving at one. This can be done through role-playing, having the child write a story about the loss, helping the child to create a good-bye ceremony, or honoring the loss in some other way (e.g., planting a tree, creating a memory book, drawing a picture of the pet, etc.).

Kyle and Jesse

Kyle's family moved from San Francisco to Santa Rosa, California, when he was 6 years old. Kyle, age 12, recalled fondly his 2-year-old terrier Jesse, who had run away from home the day that they moved. "Jesse was a really, really neat dog. She was really funny and loved to play. The day we moved, she ran off. We looked for her for but couldn't find her. Then it was time to go. We had to leave her." When asked what he thought happened to her, he said, "We figured that because she was such a great dog, someone must've found her and taken her home." When asked if he thought Jesse was with her new family, he said, "I'd like to think so. She might be dead, though."

Kyle's first pet loss occurred when he was moving to a new town where he needed to make new friends and attend a new school. He had not forgotten this loss, and he needed to share it with his friends when one of the boys was talking about his new dog. Years later, Kyle tried to resolve the loss by creating and wanting to believe the "happy-ending" story in which Jesse finds a new home, but another part of Kyle knew realistically that the dog might have died.

Children might want to keep their hope and faith alive that the pet may return. Although children should be encouraged to continue to have hope and faith, at the same time it is important that the caregiver assist the child in working through feelings of loss, abandonment, and uncertainty. A caregiver should never take away the child's hope by saying, "You need to get over this; Mittens is never going to return." Although adults might intend to help children face an inevitability rather than prolong false hope, children will arrive at their own conclusions in their own time, and they should be supported in doing so. This can best be achieved by acknowledging children's hope while supporting them through the process of slowly letting go. By the same token, caregivers should not mislead children by telling them not to grieve because the pet will most likely return. An appropriate statement is "Although I cannot promise that we will find Raina, we will do everything within our power to bring her home."

It is significant to note that there are cases in which a pet does return. However, when the uncertainty of the pet's fate endures over a long time, feelings of grief and loss arise and must be worked through. By helping children fully work through their feelings and allowing them to arrive at their own conclusions, caregivers are helping to lay a foundation children can build from as they mature and continue to make sense of the loss.

As children mature, so does their understanding of death and loss. Children will spend years thinking about the loss in an attempt to make sense of it. This is why it is so important for an adult assisting a child through a loss not to try to "fix" it. Offering a happy-ending story may appease a child at age 5, but as the child matures and intellectual capabilities change, his or her understanding and awareness of loss deepens.

Placing a Pet for Adoption

Making a decision to place a pet for adoption can be difficult, especially when children are part of the family and share a bond with the pet. There are many reasons why pet owners consider giving a pet to another family or placing it with a humane organization:

- a family member's allergies
- housing restrictions due to a recent or anticipated move;
- animal behavior problems (such as aggression toward children)
- problems in the way children in the family behave toward the pet
- a divorce, death, or birth in the family
- a drop in income
- a failure to bond with the pet
- pressure from neighbors or law enforcement (e.g., for animals who bark excessively or get loose)
- a job that requires frequent travel
- a child leaving home to attend college and the parents refuse or are unable to care for the pet
- the pet owner's terminal illness or disability[1]

Sometimes families will decide to adopt a pet without knowing what it will really be like to care for a pet or what the pet's temperament is like and how it might respond to being a part of the family. In any of these situations, choosing to place a pet for adoption is a decision that affects the entire family. Because of this, children should be included in the decision-making process. This process might include explaining to the children why the decision needs to be made and what will happen to the pet. It can also include allowing children to share their input about the pet's fate (where it will live, etc.).

Sometimes well-meaning parents might decide to remove the pet from the home when the child is away at school. When the child inquires about the pet, the parents tell the child a story about the pet's fate. I have worked with parents who told their children what I call "the farm story," in which the pet is said to have been given to a nice farmer who has lots of animals the pet can play with and lots of land for it to live on. Most of the time, children eventually question this story and as a result lose faith in their parents' truthfulness. Whatever is decided, the feelings of the children should be discussed and validated, and the caregiver should encourage them to express their grief. Allowing children to say good-bye to the pet is vital to helping them work through the loss. By encouraging a child to say good-bye and to express emotions, the caregiver acknowledges and validates the bond the child shares with the pet.

Caregivers should carefully consider what they say to children regarding the adoption. For instance, when Billy asked his parents if it was his fault that they were giving their cat Rufus to another home, his mother asked him what he meant. Billy said that his older brother had angrily told him that Rufus had to leave because Billy was allergic to cats.

Billy's mom explained to him that although they loved Rufus, they also loved Billy and that he was their first priority. She explained that they had not known that anyone in the family was allergic to cats until they adopted Rufus. She said that people could not help having allergies because it was just the way they were inside. She equated this to Billy's older brother's having to wear glasses. Billy asked her if she was angry with him for being allergic. She hugged him and told him no. She said that she was going to miss Rufus but that she would miss Billy even more if anything happened to him. She also explained this to Billy's brother and let the entire family know that any one of them could have had or developed an allergy to cats. In doing so, she was asking the family to show compassion to Billy and to understand why the decision to give the cat to another home had been made.

Because Billy's mom made it safe for Billy to approach her with his feelings, Billy was able to share his concerns without fear of being abandoned or rejected. Billy's mom was able to provide him with insight and knowledge regarding the loss. His understanding and awareness, and that of the entire family, made it easier for Billy to see that the Rufus's adoption was not his fault.

When a Parent Accidentally Kills a Pet

One of the most difficult pet losses a family can experience is when a parent accidentally kills the pet. Some of the most common ways a pet loss can occur are when pets are run over by automobiles, accidentally closed in garage doors, strangled by ropes when tethered to objects, accidentally poisoned by snail bait or rat poison, or overheated when accidentally left in direct sunlight. Parents must accept responsibility for the accident, learn from it, and assist their children through the loss. Working through this type of pet loss can include exploring feelings of blame, guilt, and anger.

The following case example involves a parent, her son, and the tragic accidental loss of a pet followed by another tragic loss several years later.

George and Daisy

George was 6 years old when his mother left his bunny Daisy in her cage in the hot sun. She was cleaning the patio and moved Daisy to what was then shade. However, as the day wore on she forgot that she had left Daisy in a new spot, and she did not check to see if the cage was still in the shade. George came home from school and discovered Daisy's lifeless body in her cage. He and his mother rushed Daisy to the veterinary hospital. The veterinarian examined Daisy with George present and pronounced her dead. George had many questions about death. The veterinarian, with George's mother's permission, patiently answered his questions. He let George listen with the stethoscope to Daisy's heart. George said that he could not hear anything. The veterinarian said it was because Daisy's heart had stopped beating, which is something that happened to all living creatures when they died.

George's mom shared her grief and guilt at having been the one to leave the cage in a sunny spot. The veterinarian acknowledged her feelings and said to her and George that it had been an accident. He said that he knew them to be very good pet owners who would not have purposely done something like this. George and his mother took Daisy's body home to bury.

A couple of months later, George brought his kitten Chloe to see the veterinarian. The veterinarian examined Chloe and talked to George about caring for his new pet. He told George that he was confident that he would be a good pet owner for Chloe because he had loved and cared for Daisy so well.

George and Chloe visited the veterinarian over the course of several years. George was a very good pet owner. When George was 12 years old, he and his mother rushed Chloe to the veterinarian. George's mother had accidentally closed Chloe in the garage door as she was driving away and had not found her until she returned home. The veterinarian pronounced Chloe dead. George's mother felt guilty and was terribly ashamed. She said that she had been responsible for Daisy's death and was now responsible for Chloe's death almost 6 years later. George was distraught and allowed his tears to flow freely. He also hugged his crying mother and told her that it was an accident, that she had loved and cared for Chloe, and that he did not blame her and did not want her to blame herself. Through their shared grief and the lessons they learned through the loss of Daisy, George and his mother were able to work through the loss of Chloe.

George learned a valuable life lesson about love and forgiveness through the loss of his pets. Through George's compassionate attitude, and the support of the family's veterinarian, George's mother learned to forgive herself and to trust herself again with the care of another family pet, obtained 6 months after the death of the Chloe.

A caregiver should never say any of the following to a child:

- "Well, that's what happens when you leave the gate open: the dog runs out and gets killed."
- "It's your fault for not feeding your guinea pig. It starved."
- "I told you that if you left your bunny's cage in the sun the bunny would die."
- "If you had really loved your bird, you would've checked to make certain the latch to the cage door was hitched."

Although all of these statements may be truthful, they are also hurtful. Blaming and placing guilt on a child only hinders the grieving process. The child knows what happened. Parents must also share in the responsibility for a pet, because children are not fully capable of caring for pets on their own until they are old enough to babysit. Even then, parents should oversee pet care and provide financially for the pet.

Caregivers working with children who have been blamed for the death of the pet should help them understand that although their actions (e.g., leaving a gate open) or inactions (e.g., not feeding a pet, not giving it water) played a role in the pet's demise, they had not intended to harm the pet. Such children need to learn to forgive themselves and others. At the pet loss support group we often talk about the gifts that come from loving and losing a pet. One gift a child can receive from such an experience is that of learning to have compassion for oneself and others. This is one of the most significant aspects of human development. To learn to love and care for others, and to love and care for oneself, is what makes us human and distinguishes us from other forms of life.

Alan Wolfelt, in his book, *Children And Grief*, eloquently discusses grief.

> In a very real sense, grief is a privilege for both children and adults, in that the capacity for deep feelings exists in a way that lower forms of life are not able to appreciate and experience. Only because we have the capacity for a loving relationship is it possible that we are able to grieve. When children are born into this world, they do not have the choice of feeling or not feeling. The capacity to feel is inevitable. However, as adults, we do have the choice as to how open and honest we will be with our children regarding the full spectrum of feelings and how committed we will be in helping both ourselves and our children in working through these feelings in a healthy, life-giving manner. As caregivers, openness and honesty are essential.

When a Child Who Has a Disability Loses a Pet

It was not that long ago that people began teaching animals to aid people with disabilities. Animals have always helped children to feel safe, secure, confident, and accepted. Sometimes, in addition, they are extensions of the child's body, acting as eyes or ears for children with disabilities. The loss of such an animal is a loss on multiple levels. A child who depends on a dog to see for him or her will have to grieve the loss of that dog while adjusting to the burden of not having that assistance. Furthermore, the child will have to bond with another seeing-eye dog, often before the process of grieving the departed dog is completed. Many times children will have to work through a multitude of feelings while making many new adjustments. When bonding with another working companion animal, they will have to learn to trust a new dog again. Children might compare the new animal with the one that died, which can bring up feelings of sadness, frustration, anger, and even fear. Children might be unwilling or unable to bond with a new animal while they are working through the loss of the old one. Complicating this is the need to assistance with their disability and bond with a new dog.

The child should be helped to understand that he or she might not bond with a new animal right away and that this is OK. No animal will ever replace the one that died. Allow the child the space in which to say good-bye and express emotion. Learning to bond and trust again are lessons of childhood that all children go through. Learning to bond and trust an animal that assists in daily living requires patience, understanding, and time. Sometimes encouraging the child to talk with the new animal about the animal that died can help to facilitate the grieving process. It also helps to facilitate a new relationship with a new dog.

Children Who Raise Dogs to Be Placed With People With Disabilities

There are animal training programs in the United States that rely on families to assist in the raising of puppies for people who have disabilities. However, asking a child to accept, love, and help raise a puppy then say good-bye to it a year later involves a kind of bonding. The family bonds with the dog and them must experience the loss of saying goodbye to it. Without good communication within the family structure, clear expectations, and participation in the process to the fullest, children are more likely to have a difficult time loving a pet and then saying good-bye to it.

One unique program that relies on volunteer families to assist in raising puppies to become working dogs that assist disabled people is Canine Companions for Independence (CCI), in Santa Rosa, California. The following case example discusses some of the issues regarding puppy raising and releasing the puppy for advanced training in the hope of it ultimately becoming a partner for a person with disabilities.

Karen, Larry, Joanne, James, and Eloise

"How could you do that to your children?" Karen, a puppy raiser for CCI, was frequently asked this question regarding her 7-year-old son James and 9-year-old daughter Joanne. Karen said that she felt she was providing her children with a wonderful learning experience. One that teaches compassion for others and selflessness. "I know it sounds corny," stated Karen, "but it's really about loving something and setting it free." She continued to say, "It's a really powerful experience."

Karen's husband Larry works for CCI. They made a decision, as a family, to raise a puppy that would be turned in to the program for advanced training, then placed with a person in a wheelchair. The puppy Eloise lived with them for a year and a half. During that time, Karen said they did their best as a family to train Eloise and love her so that she would one day be a gift for someone with disabilities. During this time the children got to see people in wheelchairs receive the dogs, that graduated from CCI, and would assist them in a variety of ways in their lives.

Karen said that they all became very attached to Eloise. They also knew that at the end of the year and a half they would be relinquishing her to CCI. The day came when they had to say good-bye to Eloise. James and Joanne said good-bye to the dog in the morning before school. Larry took Eloise to work with him, and Karen said that there were plenty of tears. However, although everyone in the family was attached to Eliose, it was a "different sort of attachment than you have with a family pet." The difference was that going into it they knew that they were going to have to say good-bye to the dog and that she would become a gift to someone who would love and care for her and benefit from her training.

Karen attributed the ability of the family to raise a CCI dog and work through the loss to communication: "You have to be really up-front about what's going to happen from the beginning." She said that the communication continued throughout the puppy-raising process with reminders that

Eloise would be leaving the home. Also, allowing children to meet people who benefited from the gift of a CCI dog helped them to see that they were performing a loving act of kindness. In addition, allowing the children to say good-bye to the dog and grieve the loss was very important in helping them to work through their feelings.

Sometimes during advance training the dogs can be chosen for breeding dogs. They can also be dropped from the program and made available for adoption. The puppy-raising family is approached to keep a breeding dog or to receive a dog for adoption.

Eloise was in the advanced training program when the decision to make her a breeding dog was made. Eloise was returned to Karen and her family. She was having her first litter of puppies when I interviewed Karen for this book. She said that she and her family were happy to have Eloise living with them. Karen also reminded that the children, although excited about the puppies, would soon be saying good-bye to them as they went to CCI puppy-raising homes. It is a process that is not without sadness and tears. However, Karen said it was a wonderful way for her children to learn that they can help make a difference in the lives of other people.

The Importance of a Pet to an Ill Child

A pet can sit for hours either on or next to a child's bed. Even very ill children may be able to stroke a pet or just take comfort in its presence. One adult pet owner shared with me the time when she was 12 years old and in a body cast. She was very sad that she could not play with her friends or participate in activities that she had enjoyed prior to her surgery. Her sister brought her a kitten. "That kitten changed my life," she said. The kitten would curl up on her body cast and snuggle under her chin as she lay in bed. She was able to stroke the kitten, talk to it, and even play with it, despite her limited capacity to move. For some ill children, just knowing a pet has come to greet them will help them to temporarily

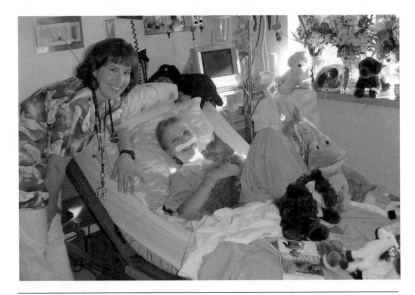

Figure 4.1 Animals bring immeasurable comfort to children in the hospital.

forget their discomfort and take joy in watching the animal. Animals accept children at face value. They do not pass judgment, and they do not fear seeing children hooked up to IV tubes and monitors or smelling hospital smells. Pets do not ask children questions. They are there for ill children as unconditional presences that can sometimes elicit smiles and offer tactile stimulation. Children who are experiencing an illness should be allowed contact with their pet unless there is some medical reason why the pet might be detrimental to their health.

Children Who Share Illnesses With Their Pets

Although I have yet to work with a child who has had an illness similar to his or her pet's illness, I have worked with adults and families who struggled with caring for human and animal family members simultaneously afflicted with cancer. Susan Chernak McElory, author of *Animals as Teachers and Healers,* wrote about losing her dog to cancer and then being faced with it herself.[2] She discussed the unique gifts that her dog bestowed on her and included testimonies from other pet owners.

Pets can teach us to live in the moment. They can teach us to not hold a grudge, be happy for what we have, play hard, sleep well, and be grateful for the food bestowed on us. They teach us to love with our whole heart, be loyal, and forgive easily and readily. All of these lessons are gifts that children can apply to everyday life, and they take on even more importance when children are faced with challenges such as illness. Many ill animals teach their caregivers that they enjoy life as much as they possibly can, they rest quietly when they cannot play, and they continue to express love and affection for those who care for them. In my work as a pet loss grief therapist, many adult pet owners have shared with me lessons about living with an illness. One of the most profound lessons a terminally ill client shared with me was that her dog taught her how to die with dignity. These are lessons or gifts that children can experience from sharing an illness with a pet.

McElory wrote that the loss of her father was the first (human) immediate death in her family that she had to cope with. She wrote,

> Yet the devastation of its impact had been made more bearable for me by a seemingly endless, beloved string of animal companions, all long ago loved and long gone. Through them I had learned how to grieve and how to let go. In the solemnity of countless backyard burials, I discovered the value of ritual and altar making. Holding my dying pets and feeling life float way from them like some luminous fog, I came to know through touch alone the glaring distinction between life and nonlife, that incomprehensible moment when a living being exhales into death. Living beyond the deaths of my animal companions, I learned that time softens the hurt and sweetens the memories. And as my animal companions have returned to live again in my dreams and in my heart, I am reminded over and over that love doesn't know death.[3]

Animals have much to offer children regarding life, love, and loss. They are quiet, soulful teachers to whom children can easily and readily relate and bond. Children may not even realize all the gifts that sharing a life with an animal bestows on them until they are adults, as McElory discovered.

Conclusion

Pets do not die through euthanasia only. They might run away from home, be stolen, be tragically killed, be placed for adoption, be lost in custody battles, or become victims of accidental death. Because of the variety of ways a pet loss can occur, it is necessary to be familiar with many types of losses and ways in which to assist a child through special or unique losses. Regardless of the circumstances surrounding the loss, the caregiver must work closely with the child to ascertain the meaning of the loss and the specific emotions the child attaches to it. For example, a caregiver might assume that a child feels guilty over the death of a pet that was hit by a car and killed because the child neglected to latch a gate. However, the child may not make this connection and feel sad and angry that the pet has died. He or she might have many questions about the loss, rather than feel guilty about how it occurred.

In other cases, as I mentioned in this chapter, children do feel responsible and guilty for their roles, real or imagined, in the loss of their pets. The caregiver must realistically define the child's role in the pet's death. If the child perceives himself or herself in some way responsible for the death, the initial focus should be to alleviate the guilt with which the child is struggling.

Pets can be good medicine for an ill child. Ill pets can teach children life lessons about being compassionate, living in the moment, fighting for life, and even dying. However a pet loss occurs, it is important for caregivers to learn what the loss means to the child and how the child perceives the loss and the role of the child, if any, in the pet's demise.

5
WHEN TO ADOPT ANOTHER PET

When one door closes, another opens. But we often look so regretfully upon the closed door that we don't see the one that has opened for us.

—Alexander Graham Bell

The problem with hearts is that they break, and a broken heart brings pain. It takes courage to learn to trust again and to have faith to learn to love again. Having both courage and faith is an integral part of being human and of maturing. When someone or something we love dies, the pain that comes with it can seem unbearable. To learn to be willing to love again and to let our hearts feel deeply for another pet is an act of faith and courage. Children need to learn to have faith and to be taught to believe that although life seems sad and lonely after a loss, one day soon they will again feel happiness.

Children vary greatly in their responses to bonding with another pet after one has died. Some start discussing the possibility of a new pet right after one has died. Others state that they are not so certain they want another pet. There are lessons in grief. Children of any age should know that there is a period of mourning that follows a death. Those we have loved and lost can never be replaced, and the unique bond that was shared cannot be replaced either.

Children can learn that it is OK to want to develop deep feelings for another pet, and it is also OK to wait before deciding to adopt again. Children can also be taught to respect other family members' feelings regarding death. I remember that within a single week, two of my family's rabbits died. Although both rabbits were loved, one was much more a part of the family than the other one had been. My 11-year-old daughter wanted to get another rabbit right away because we no longer had a bunny. However, the rest of the family was not ready to bond with another rabbit. We discussed the reasons that our bunnies were special, significant, and unique. I explained to her that I needed time to grieve and heal after the loss of our rabbits before I could learn to love another one again and enjoy the special attributes that he or she would bring to our family. My daughter accepted this and respected our decision to wait. She learned that although you can fill the void of not having a pet by adopting another pet, the void in your heart takes time to heal. She also learned that it would not be fair to herself, other family members, or another pet if we were to adopt before we all felt ready to do so.

If children view pets as replaceable, they might try to use replacement as a way to avoid grieving. Grieving a loss is natural, necessary, and healthy. Children need to be taught this, as it will help them to cope with future losses. Children who do not mourn the loss of a pet can have difficulty bonding with another. They might look to the pet to fill the void the loss has left and expect the new pet to be like the one they lost. They might become angry, irritated, and unhappy with the new pet for not behaving in the same manner or having similar traits as the pet that is gone. Often these new pets are neglected, abandoned, relinquished to humane agencies, or given away, which can result in even more grief, and feelings of sadness, despair, anger, and depression can still appear.

By the same token, children who are grieving should have their grief respected by the adults who care for them. Although it can be difficult for a parent to understand the bond

a child had with a goldfish, it is important that the adult validate and respect the child's grief and loss. I remember watching an episode of *America's Funniest Home Videos* in which
two little girls held a funeral for their fish. Part of the ritual of
the funeral was flushing the fish down the toilet. The girls
made several attempts to place the fish in the toilet and then
flush it. Each time they burst into tears and backed away
from doing it. The parents videotaping the scene laughed, as
did the audience watching it. The video won a prize, but the
look on the little girls' faces said it all. They were not happy
they had won. Something they loved had died and the adults
in their lives saw only the humor in the all-too-familiar situation of flushing a dead fish down a toilet.

In *Pet Loss: A Thoughtful Guide for Adults and Children*,
Neiburg and Fischer wrote, "Stifling one's emotions by invest-
ing energy and love in another pet does not eliminate grief; it
merely pushes it into the background and delays its resolution. The sense of loss may take years to dissipate—or it may
never disappear."[1]

Caregivers should consider and discuss the following questions with older children, and consider them with younger children, when the subject of adopting another pet is brought up:

1. Are you ready for the responsibility of a new pet?
2. Have you worked through and resolved your loss?
3. Are you open to loving and caring for a new pet?
4. Will you be able to view the new pet as a unique and
    special being?
5. Do you feel as if family members and friends are pres-
    suring you into getting another pet?
6. Why do you want to adopt another pet?
7. Do you realize that a new pet will be very different from
    the one that is gone?

Although acquiring a new pet can be therapeutic and healing, it is important to work through the loss fully before jump-
ing into a new relationship.

Younger children seem to work through their losses more quickly and more fully than older children. One reason can be found in the child's cognitive age. Very young children have limited understanding of death and loss. Older children are more intellectually stimulated by a loss, and as such can think more deeply about their feelings, circumstances surrounding the loss, and their involvement, if any, in the loss. Also, older children have more layered and busy lives in which other issues can factor into their grieving. They also might be continuing to work on past losses as their understanding matures and deepens.

A younger child might be ready much sooner than an older one to adopt another pet. Older children may have to contend with issues a younger child might not consider, such as loyalty conflicts. Some children can feel that bonding with another pet is an act of disloyalty toward the one that is gone. They become irritated by a younger child's insistence on getting another pet. Children who are given a new pet too quickly might feel that their loyalty lies with the deceased pet, or they might believe that their parents did not really love the lost animal. Unfortunately, it is not uncommon for young children to wonder how quickly their parents might replace them if they were to die. These issues can best be worked through if children are encouraged to share their beliefs, emotions, and expectations about adopting a new pet when deciding about whether, and when, to get another pet.

Children should be taught that deciding to bond with another pet is a family decision. Each family member should be able to speak freely about his or her feelings regarding the loss and the acquisition of a new pet. Here are some guidelines from *Pet Loss and Human Emotion: Guiding Clients Through Grief* regarding successful bonding with a new pet:[2]

1. Remember that the decision to acquire another pet does not represent disloyalty to a deceased pet.
2. Do not expect the pet to become an instant family member. Give the relationship time to develop.

3. Bring the new pet home when things are calm. Holidays are not the best time to introduce new pets into the family.
4. Do not expect the new pet to be like the deceased pet.
5. Encourage children to allow their feelings for their previous pet to surface. If their new pet is doing something that reminds them of their previous pet, encourage them to express the feelings that come along with this.
6. Allow other family members to adjust to the new pet and bond in their own time.

In their book *The Human-Animal Bond and Grief,* Lagoni et al. wrote that some pet owners take comfort in talking with their new pets about their old pets.[3] They suggested showing the new pet a photo of a deceased pet as a means of introducing the two. Sometimes children do this naturally. One little girl who had a photo of her cat who died a 3 years prior to her getting another kitten often showed the photo to the new kitten and told him about the cat who died. This child had found a way to continue to work through the previous loss, and she had found a very healthy tool for working through future losses.

Trying to fix a grieving child's loss by getting a replacement animal should never be done. Offering a stuffed toy or helping the child to create a scrapbook or some other kind of memory book are better ways to help the child to cope with and work through the loss. Showing an interest in attending the funeral of a pet that died and participating in one also greatly aids a child in saying good-bye. (I discuss further the importance of saying good-bye in chapter 6.)

When a child is ready to adopt a pet, the entire family should participate in the decision-making process. There are many ways to obtain a new pet. If a pet is to be adopted from an animal shelter or rescue organization, children should be prepared ahead of time for what they might see and experience. Often children feel sorry for the pets in cages and want to take them all home. Sometimes if the children are young, parents might first visit a shelter and arrange for one or two pets they are considering for adoption to be shown to the children in a private room. This helps to avoid the overwhelming emotion that might come with seeing so many animals in need of a good home.

The pet's temperament and suitability for the environment in which it is to live should be taken into consideration as well. If the pet is a mixed breed, the qualities and behavioral traits of those breeds should be known and considered prior to the adoption. Some breeds of pets may not be the best choice for interacting with children. The pet's health should be checked prior to the adoption. A parent should consider taking the pet to the veterinarian prior to bringing it home. All of these things will help to avoid another loss in having to return a pet that is unhealthy or difficult to handle.

Conclusion

The decision to adopt a pet should always be a family decision. A pet should not be adopted until all members of the family feel ready to share their lives with one again.

Children should be included in the decision-making process. Educating children about the types of animals that make the best pets for specific family considerations is wise prior to choosing the pet. Discussing what is expected of each family member regarding the pet's care and contracting for it with older children will help to ensure that the adoption process is successful. Exploring adoption options ahead of time and researching different breeds will also help to provide a smooth transition. Taking the pet to the veterinarian prior to bringing it home is wise to make certain the pet is healthy. In addition, talking to the new pet about the pet that is gone can be therapeutic for all family members. Children should feel free to discuss the differences they note between the new pet's behavior and the behavior of the one that is gone. This helps the children to understand that the newest family member is a separate, unique animal, as was the one that is now gone, and is in no way a replacement.

Taking time to fully explore the adoption process and include each person's input will help to make bonding with another animal a happy transition. Learning to respect each family member regarding a period of mourning and to `support each other in choosing to love a pet again is healthy and teaches the child about loss and love.

6
SAYING GOOD-BYE

Even when walking through the dark valley of death I will not
be afraid, for you are close beside me, guarding, guiding all the
way.

—Psalms 23:4

Believing in something, having faith, and feeling loved are
key factors in working through a loss. Some children may be
encouraged to believe in a higher power. Whatever a family's
beliefs, the important factor in assisting a child through a
loss is support. Immediate family support is ideal. Extended
support from caregivers can ease the suffering of the child
and significantly aid in the healing process. We all need to
know that we are not alone in our grief. Children especially
need to know that someone is there walking beside them. A
bond of love, in any form, should be acknowledged, validated,
and honored. Children can be assisted in creating ways to
remember their pets and to say good-bye to them. Sometimes the good-bye is forever (as in the death of a pet); other
times a good-bye is only for now (as in a temporary adoption,
or when a pet leaves home and the pet returns). In either
case, a loss occurs and the child can benefit from creating
ways in which the life shared with the pet is honored.

If You Love Something, Set It Free: The Mitchell Family's Pigeon

The Mitchell family shared this poignant story about saying good-bye. Pidgie was an orphaned baby pigeon discovered at the ice arena where the Mitchell girls, Carmen and Antonia, skate. A pigeon had built a nest inside the arena and laid two eggs that hatched. Carmen and Antonia discovered one of the baby pigeons on the ice. They took her home, and with the help of their mom, Adele, they nursed her back to health. They named the little bird Pidgie and provided her with loving care. Over time, the little bird grew big and was no longer content to stay in her cage. Adele and her husband, Tom, talked to their daughters about setting Pidgie free.

They did not want their bird to fly away; however, they knew that as a wild creature she would not be content to live caged. With much sadness they ceremoniously let the little bird go. The bird flew to the top of their play structure and there she stayed. Concerned that Pidgie might not know how to seek food and shelter, the Mitchells placed Pidgie's cage, filled with food and water, on top of the play structure with the little door latched open. Pidgie was content to fly around the yard and move in and out of her cage. Sometimes the bird would land on Adele's head and say hello. Other times she would perch on the kitchen windowsill and peer inside the family's home as Adele washed dishes.

One day the little bird flew away. She did not return. The family was sad to lose their special bird. They hoped that she had survived and found a flock to join. A few months later they knew that what they hoped for had happened. Pidgie returned to the yard with a flock of pigeons. The birds eagerly ate the food the Mitchells placed on top of the play structure for them. Pidgie flew down and landed on Adele's head, as she had done many times in the past. The family came outside to visit with Pidgie. They stroked and kissed the bird and then watched as she once again flew away.

It has been 4 years since Pidgie first came to live at the Mitchells' house. She still comes to visit a few times a year and often brings members of her flock. Adele said that recently Pidgie perched herself on the windowsill and stared inside. Adele came out and Pidgie flew up to the cage on top of the play structure and back toward Adele. Adele watched as the bird did this a few times. Adele said that she thought Pidgie was trying to tell her something, and Pidgie was. She wanted food.

Adopting Pidgie, loving her, and then letting her go was a powerful lesson for the entire family, said Adele, especially for the girls. They learned to love unselfishly. Letting her go was an act of faith and hope that she would one day return and, most important, belief that she would be able to survive on her own.

Although we cannot always be with the things we love, we can keep them close to us in our hearts. Although the Mitchells never wanted to lose Pidgie, they knew that they had to let her go for her to continue to thrive and live a full life. They also learned that in letting her go they had not lost Pidgie forever. Pidgie remembered them and continues to return to them.

Sometimes the hardest thing in life is to say good-bye and trust that someone we love will return to us. Although there are no guarantees, there is always hope that we will be reunited with those we love, and we can have faith by believing that they will be all right.

When our good-byes are permanent, a memorial helps to honor those we love and will never forget. Creating a memorial garden in which a plaque is placed in honor of the pet can help a child to feel that he or she is doing something beautiful and heartfelt for the deceased pet. It can be therapeutic to work side by side with a parent or other children in bringing new life to a patch of dirt in honor of the love that was shared with the pet.

Children have created beautiful collages and shared them with other people at the pet loss support group I lead. A collage can assist children in remembering special times shared with the pet that is now gone. It can provide an opportunity for children to talk about the pet and the feelings that were experienced, as well as what their pet meant to them.

Some of the most poignant examples of feelings around loss have been illustrated in drawings. One little girl drew a picture of a dog, King, that belonged to one of the workmen who spent several months working on her house. Every day the dog would come to work with him and the little girl would play with the dog. One day the workman came alone and told the girl that the dog had died. That night she went up to her room and drew a picture of the dog wearing angel wings. The dog was sitting on a cloud. Below the cloud was a drawing of the workman. The little girl wrote, "King is looking down on you now making sure that you are okay."

A child might decide to wear the cat's collar as a bracelet to feel close to a cat that has died. Some children choose to cuddle or sleep with the pet's bedding. One woman shared that she saved her dog's blue collar and wore it as a garter—for something blue—under her wedding gown in honor of the dog with whom she had grown up.

Holding funerals for even the tiniest of pets is honoring established rituals for mourning the deceased. It may seem unreasonable or even silly to a parent to bury a guppy, but to the child who experienced the loss, it honors the bond shared and allows the child to say good-bye. Many children like to bury the pet's body or ashes so that they can have a place to visit and talk to their deceased pet. Many funerals have taken place under my 10-year-old daughter's "baby tree" throughout her growing up. The baby tree is a tree that was planted on the day that she was born. She made the decision to bury her pets under the tree that started growing when she did. It is a place for her to sit and visit and talk to the many birds,

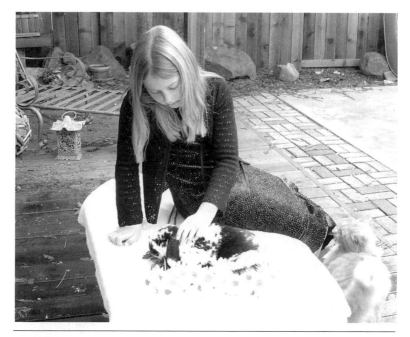

Figure 6.1 Savannah holds a funeral to say goodbye to her rabbit Harry.

fish, and mice that have been buried under the tree. We have discussed how the animal's body returns to the earth and feeds the tree, thus helping it to grow and blossom. In this small ritual, a circle of life has been concretely established in her mind as a way of helping her to understand life and death, loving and letting go.

Letting go takes trust. Rituals for saying good-bye help children to establish trust in those around them, thus providing them with the ability to release the loss and move on. It is often shocking for a child to learn that life is not permanent and that sooner or later we all die.

In creating mourning rituals, we teach children that life and grief are honored and respected. Children can learn that the ability to give and receive love is one of the most fundamentally important aspects of living. Memorializing something that we loved allows us to honor the bond shared and maintain a touchstone in working through the loss. I have often felt in my grief work that the memorial should be left up to those who are living, and that people who know they are going to die and request that no funeral or celebration of life service take place are robbing those who have to go on without them of an important ritual for saying good-bye and thus working through the loss.

Children are often very good at coming up with their own rituals for death. Children might want to lay out the pet's body, pet it, or ask questions about the changes in it from when life was present to how the pet's body feels now that life is gone. They might look into the pet's eyes. They might decide to form a circle around it, say prayers, talk about its life, or just cry. Other children might decide that they do not want to do any of these things, because they feel very angry or disengaged with the process. Allow the child to express the funeral, but do not deny a child the right to say good-bye either.

Burial Options

There are many ways in which to honor a pet's body. The most common ways are through burial on the pet owner's property or in a pet cemetery and through cremation. When a pet is cremated, the ashes can be scattered at the pet memorial park or returned to the pet owner in a small cedar box. Children might want to bury the ashes or keep the box in a prominent place at home. One child placed a photo of him and his dog on top of the cedar box that held the dog's ashes. Another child helped her mom scatter the ashes over the rose garden in their backyard. One family placed their pet's ashes in a papier-mâché pillow, placed it in the river they used to in play with their dog, and said their final good-byes as they watched the pillow float on the water and out to sea.

A Child's Pet Cemetery

One child, Kristy, shared with me her ritual for burying her pets. She created a pet cemetery on her property. For each grave, she would find three large stones. One had to be flat on one surface; this one would be placed on top of the others

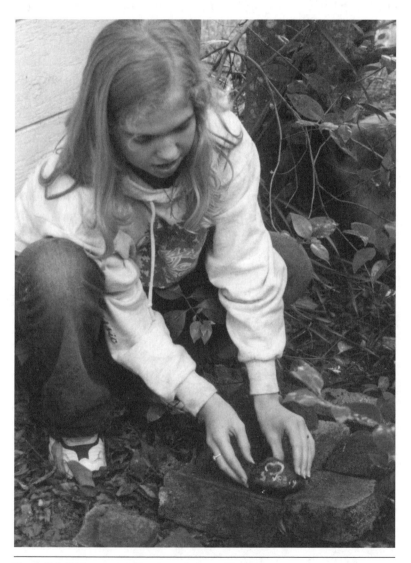

Figure 6.2 Kristy arranges the stones in her pet cemetery.

as a marker. On the flat stone she would use "rainbow paint" to write the pet's name on the stone. She would place silk flowers on the new graves "because they last longer." Her mother said that Kristy often lovingly attended her pet cemetery in the spring, removing any weeds and debris. Kristy shared with me her annoyance at having an unwelcomed visitor. A raccoon visited her cemetery and toppled the stones placed on her pet's graves.

Children might choose to write a poem or story about their pet and the life that was shared. They can send little presents to go with the pet's body to be buried or cremated. The most important thing a caregiver can do for a grieving child is to acknowledge the grief, let the child know that he or she is there for him or her, and allow the child to say good-bye in the way that he or she desires.

Sometimes pet owners want to keep tangible reminders of the life they shared with their pets. Many veterinary hospitals now make a paw print for the pet's owner to keep. Other families make their own prior to the pet's death and use them as stepping-stones in a garden in which they scatter the pet's ashes. Sometimes a veterinarian will inquire as to whether the family would like to keep a clipping of the pet's fur. Often pet owners fill a lovely box with the pet's mementos (e.g., favorite toy, blanket, collar and tags, photos, clipping of fur). These are ways of staying connected to the pet and keeping remembrances of the life shared. A box or photo album can be tucked away until a child is ready to revisit the objects.

Flushing fish down a toilet might even be appropriate if the child chooses to say good-bye in this way. The important thing to remember is that the way in which a child chooses to say good-bye honors and respects the child's grief and validates the loss.

The Funeral

Being invited to attend a funeral a child is holding for a beloved pet is always an honor. One such funeral was for Froggie the frog. Froggie lived for 6 years in an aquarium in the kitchen of Taylor, Samantha, and Seth. After he died, Froggie was lovingly wrapped in an old dishtowel and placed to rest under a cherry blossom tree in the backyard. The tree was in full bloom, and many blossoms were on it and scattered around the ground below. Many of the children's small pets were buried here. The oldest child, Seth, at age 14 years, told his younger siblings Samantha and Taylor how Froggie's body would become part of the earth and feed the tree, as their other pets had done.

Seth and Taylor dug a shallow grave near the base of the tree. Samantha unwrapped the towel and laid Froggie on a bed of blossoms she sprinkled in the grave. Seth and Taylor each offered a fond memory of Froggie. Taylor talked about how tiny Froggie was when they first got him and how much he had grown. Seth remembered feeding him every morning before he left for school. He remembered how much fun it was to watch Froggie swim in the aquarium. Samantha cried and talked about how many pets of theirs had died this past year. They had endured five other losses that included fish, rabbits, and a bird. She told Froggie that he would be with their other pets and that they would all be together.

Seth and Taylor dropped handfuls of dirt on the grave. Samantha placed a shiny rock on top of the grave. She stayed at the grave site after Taylor and Seth left. Samantha cried a few more tears and then stood up. She looked at the tree and said that Froggie's body was now feeding the tree. Froggie's body was going to be a part of the tree and the blossoms that would come each spring, and he would live on through the tree.

The Therapeutic Benefits of Reaching Out to Other Children

Just keeping cherished items might not be enough to begin to work through a loss. People often need to feel as if they are doing something to help others. Baking cakes, taking flowers to honor the deceased, writing letters of condolences, and attending funerals not only help the person who has been affected directly by the loss but also help those who love and care for the person who is grieving. Children are no different. They need to know that they are helping someone they love who is in pain. They have a great desire to know that they can do something for that person. They might want to help other family members who are grieving. Doing so can also be a way to help them work through their own pain.

Although the following example includes the use of stuffed toy animals and does not address the specific concerns of a pet death, I chose to include this example because it demonstrates the importance of feeling empowered by doing something in working through a loss. In this example, the loss is of the feeling of security.

Loss occurs in our society on many levels. When the World Trade Center towers were hit and the Pentagon attacked on September 11, 2001, in the United States, even children who did not live on or near the East Coast were affected by the loss, devastation, and destruction. Many children saw the attack on television or heard about it over the radio. Others learned about it from friends or by overhearing adults talk. Children who were not immediately affected had fears; they not only had concerns for their own safety but also had concerns for the people and the children who were directly affected by the attacks.

One of the most powerful life lessons children can learn is to know that they are not alone and that a common thread of empathy binds us all.

United We Stand

When 9/11 happened, it was back-to-school night at my children's elementary school in California. Most of the artwork from children that week depicted the attacks on the World Trade Center's twin towers. Instead of ignoring the children's fears or telling them that it was just something that happened far, far away, the school organized a teddy bear drive. The elementary school contacted another elementary school located near the Pentagon. Some of the children there had parents who worked at the Pentagon. Each child at the California elementary school brought a new stuffed toy to school. They wrote messages of love, hope, and concern on index cards and tied them with ribbon around the stuffed toys. There was a ceremony held at the California school in which the children carried their stuffed toys with heartfelt messages and placed them in boxes to be mailed to the other school. They sang songs, and a paper flag of the United States made of each child's handprint was held up at the ceremony. The principal and teachers talked about faith, hope, and love. The ceremony was videotaped and sent along with the stuffed toys to the school on the East Coast. The children were shown on a map of the United States where the attacks had occurred and where their gifts were going. Teachers began corresponding with the teachers at the other school, and they established pen pals.

I included here some of the e-mail responses received by the California school in regard to the teddy bear drive. The California children felt empowered by the ritual to help to make a difference in the lives of other children who had endured a powerful loss. Although no one from the school on the East Coast lost an immediate family member, the parents poignantly describe their loss of feeling safe. The California children felt better knowing that children thousands of miles across the country were thinking of them and cared for them.

Out of loss and tragedy children can learn powerful lessons of faith and hope and that they have the ability to overcome bad things, work through their fears, and unite with others. Not only did these children learn that they can help to make a difference to others who are grieving but they also learned that they are never alone in their feelings and that there are adults who care for them who will help them work through a loss.

One parent wrote about the gift of a stuffed mouse to her son:

You have no idea how much your gift to my child made me feel. I first heard about the project from Connor [her son], and thought, "What a wonderful idea." All people around the world were affected by the events of September 11, and we were very lucky to not have lost family members. The man who lives next door to us works in the Pentagon, and came home very late, and very sooty that Tuesday night. He was, by happenstance, unhurt. It was a scary time for us.

Before "Bouse" (the stuffed toy he received) came home with Connor, I found myself crying at various times during the day, driving, shopping, working—wherever. I felt so disconnected. When Connor came home with Bouse, it caused me to turn the corner. Your thoughtfulness, caring, and actually taking action to help us heal was such a gift. Thank you so much.

Connor carried Bouse in his backpack for a week. Bouse had his head-poking out the zipper top, and could see everyone. Connor is a 5th grader, is 4 foot 11, and is over the charts for size of young people his age. The difference Bouse made in his life was to allow him to finish not only grieving for a way of life that used to be, but to complete with what happened. If another event happens, it does. The difference revolves around who we are in the matter.

What I got from your gift was that virtually every generation has faced a cataclysmic event. This does not mean that we can't be happy. It means we have the opportunity to show how great we can be. Like your family did by getting Bouse for Connor.

I remember when I was a child, practicing for the end of the world. I could never figure out why I wanted to spend the end of the earth under my desk! And that is what I feel now. I am not living my life under a desk—I am living out loud.

Our family took a trip to my parents' house to Massachusetts this past weekend. We drove past the Pentagon, and New York City to get there, and there they were (and weren't). Well—we had the best weekend we could have had—and we didn't do anything! We laughed, ate great food, were in awe of the changing trees, and played with my parents' latest puppy that they raise for Fidelco—a Guide Dog Organization for blind people. The best part was to have our family together laughing.

Thanks for your generosity, and caring—you have changed my life.

Another parent wrote about the difference the schoolchildren made by reaching out to her children during this time of tragedy:

I am the mother of two children who attend school in Lake Ridge, VA. Today was a very special day at our school. This afternoon when school was dismissed, all the children came out smiling and carrying stuff animals. How I wish I had a camera so that I could share with you all the smiling faces.

Your school's thoughtfulness has touched us greatly. My daughter had named her "new friend" Rosa. She has spoken all evening about the nice children in [Santa Rosa] California.

Monday of this week, it was necessary for myself and my children to drive pass the Pentagon. It was the first time the children had seen the building since 9/11. I had to try and explain how people can hate us even though they do not know us. How wonderful it was today to talk about how people care even though they do not know us personally. Thank you for bringing happiness to my children and all the other children at our elementary.

A mother shared how the stuffed toy helped her daughter through a difficult time:

All of us in the area are saddened and shocked at recent events just as the rest of the world is. Just because people don't live nearby certainly doesn't mean they weren't affected in the same ways we were. I work 12 miles from the Pentagon now and could see the smoke out of my office window on September 11th and lost two friends to the tragedy. Thank goodness Emily [her daughter] didn't know either of them. As I'm sure you know, it's difficult to try to explain to a 7-year-old why this happened, especially if I have no idea myself. All of the schools were closed up in this area when word got out and other than being totally broken as to what happened, about all we could tell both of our children was that they would remember that day for the rest of their lives and they would read about it in history as they went through school.

Emily received the following letter:

Dear friend,

I am very sorry about this accident that happened. I think about you all day. I hope you are okay.

Love,
Leslie

I'm not sure who was touched more by the letter, Emily or me. Anyway, it has touched this whole family, and it is wonderful how other people think of those affected when something tragic happens. Thank you again and please express Ashton's thanks to the students who took the time to show others here they care.

Barry and the Doctors

Children need to know that they can make a difference in the lives of others. Helping others can be therapeutic and can help a child move through the grief continuum from a place of helplessness to empowerment. Helping a child to write a letter, make a card, or give a stuffed animal to another child that is grieving also teaches a child to have empathy and compassion for others. Children who have experienced a loss can take their grief and do something positive to help other animals in honor of their pet that died or is missing. They might decide to volunteer at a shelter, foster a pet, assist another child in finding his or her missing pet, run a pet-sitting business, walk a dog for an elderly neighbor, or attend a funeral of a friend who is burying a pet. In addition, as I mentioned earlier, children can reach out and make a difference with other losses too.

One 13-year-old boy, Barry, decided to honor his mother at his bar mitzvah. His mother had died from breast cancer when he was 7 years old. His father was a physician at a local hospital and had remarried. Barry's stepmother discovered that she had breast cancer and went through treatment when Barry was 11 years old. Barry wanted to do something that would honor his mother and help his stepmother. Barry, with the help of his father's colleagues, hosted a fund-raiser for the breast cancer center at the hospital where his father worked. He met with a local restaurant and hired a band to perform at the event. More than 350 members of the local medical community came out to support Barry's fund-raiser and had fun doing it too. Barry was able to greet and meet many of the people who supported his event who told him what a wonderful thing he was doing on behalf of both his moms. He also raised more than $10,000 for the center. He was able to honor the life that he shared with his mother and at the same time do something that would benefit his step-mother and other patients at the breast cancer center.

Children can feel very empowered in their grief when they decide to do something that helps others. Children who have lost a pet might decide to do something that benefits a local animal shelter or rescue center. Learning to reach out and help others during a time of loss helps children to know that they are not alone, their efforts are supported, and their loss is validated and that positive actions not only can help others but also can help them to feel good about themselves.

Conclusion

All of us, especially children, need to know that we are not alone in our grief. Reading stories about loss, creating art-work representing feelings of loss, writing in a journal, and creating a story about the life shared with the pet are ways of helping a child to validate the bond shared with the pet and work through the grief. Encouraging children to reach out to other children who have experienced a loss not only helps to teach them compassion and to have empathy but also allows them to connect with other children who have loved and lost pets. Encouraging the use of rituals for saying good-bye to a pet that has died or is missing honors the life shared with the pet and validates the child's grief and depth of feelings for the pet.

7

COMPLICATED GRIEF RESPONSE TO PET LOSS

This is what [a partnership] really means: Helping one another to reach the full status of being persons, responsible beings who do not run away from life.

—Paul Tournier

In assisting children through a loss, there is a partnership that develops among the therapist, child, and adult caregivers. It is through this successful partnership, one based on mutual respect and understanding, that a grieving child can best be assisted through the process of grieving.

Most often, children will successfully work through a loss and find the support they need to continue to integrate the experience into their lives as their level of awareness and cognition grows. However, sometimes the loss of a pet may trigger unusual, intense responses in children. Normal grief responses, when carried to an extreme, can manifest in maladaptive coping mechanisms and require timely, effective crisis intervention to prevent the child's progression into self-destructive behavior. When grief responses are extreme, children will need more support, interventions, and sometimes medication to help them through a difficult time in their lives.

The despair that can accompany the loss of a companion animal can be as intense and painful for the child as the loss of a human family member or friend would be. As such, the loss must be acknowledged and validated if any intervention is to succeed.

There are many therapies to use in working with children (discussed in chapter 8). A therapist can incorporate a few different types or focus on one. With any type of therapy, the therapist should access the vulnerability of the child based on the child's cognitive age, previous losses, and degree of attachment to the pet and what it represented in the child's life. The first step is to take a thorough history from the parents or caregivers and then to spend time with the child and ask leading questions and listen carefully to responses. Therapeutic interventions with children are tailored to the children's level of understanding and their belief systems regarding death; this will vary with age and experience.

In assessing a child, gather as much information as possible from the adult caregivers. These caregivers can include parents, guardians, grandparents, older siblings, teachers, day care providers, and the child. Listen and watch for red flags. Red flags include divorce; a history of emotional or physical abuse, or both, and neglect; drug abuse; a death in the family (other than the death of the pet); previous history of depression or anxiety disorders; foster care; and adoption. Also assess for successes or failures in school, a peer support system, spiritual beliefs, other pets at home, other pet losses, sleep disturbance, suicide in the family, lack of interest in things previously enjoyed, bed-wetting, angry outbursts, eating disorders, attachment disorders, trauma experienced (if any), sexual abuse, rape, withdrawal, and isolation. The best predictor of future behavior is past behavior. For example, a child who has previously responded to major stressors with self-destructive behavior would be likely to respond similarly when faced with new stressors, such as the loss of a beloved pet. This becomes even more likely in the absence of love and nurturing.

A skilled therapist should look for areas where losses have overlapped, turning a simple grief response into one that is compounded by multiple losses that might threaten to overwhelm the child's coping skills. The best predictor of the how the child ultimately works through this loss is how the child has dealt with losses in the past (these losses might include divorce, a move, loss of a parent, loss of a best friend, change of schools, other pet losses, etc.).

After you have gathered information about the child's past history and current situation and established the meaning of the loss to the child, you need to explore the red flag areas thoroughly. Such exploration requires patience and effective listening skills, as children are not as forthcoming with their emotions as adults. It can take a while to establish rapport and trust with a child. A child, especially a very young child, might not be able to put his or her emotions into words, and other forms of therapy, such as art and play therapy, can be introduced.

Assessing the Child's Strengths

It also is important to assess strengths because your therapeutic interventions are going to focus on maximizing the child's strengths to see him or her through the loss. Strengths can include success in sports, positive peer relationships, academic success, loving and supportive adult caregivers, personal accomplishments, and healthy emotions. Once you have identified red flags and defined the child's strengths, you can plan therapeutic interventions.

For children experiencing a first loss, the role of the therapist is to help them to understand and accept the permanency of the loss while instilling hope. Most children will learn to love again and have other opportunities to do so. With teenagers, it is important to remember that what is their "whole life" on a Monday can completely change by Thursday. With a young child, a day can seem endless. When working with children, it is important to help them understand that feelings of anger, guilt, hopelessness, despair, and loneliness do not last forever. Explain to them that there is a beginning (often shock, denial), a middle (anger, guilt, sadness, dysphoria—carried to the extreme, depression), and an end (resolution) to the grieving process and that you will work with them to help them through all of these stages.

Denial

Denial is typically the first response to experiencing the loss of a pet. Denial is a coping mechanism that cushions the mind against the sudden shock it has received. Denial can last 24 hours, or go on longer. If denial persists for an extended period of time, in the face of overwhelming proof of the animal's demise, the therapist will need to sensitively resolve the fact of the pet's death. For example, a young child might exhibit magical thinking, expressing a belief that the pet will come back to life or wake up from sleeping or believing that he or she will discover the pet at the door. Care must be taken to slowly to remove the child's barriers to understanding the permanency of the pet's death. Once the child is able to accept the finality of death, then the child will be able to progress through the grieving process. Very young children (younger than the age of 5 years) who are not cognitively able to understand the finality of death might not be in denial, but they might need repeated reminders that the pet will not be returning.

Mason and Petey

One 4-year-old child, Mason, repeatedly exhumed the body of his pet bird Petey to reassure himself that Petey was not alive. It was his attempt to understand and cope with his loss. After a week of digging up Petey, Mason's mother told him that he could no longer do this because Petey's body would be in a condition that they would not want to remember. She talked to her son about remembering Petey's sitting on his perch chirping and how much they enjoyed him while he was alive. Mason seemed to accept this explanation and his mother's suggestion to plant flowers on top of Petey's grave. While planting the flowers, Mason's mother explained that the nuturients in the soil, which have been nourished, in part, by Petey's body, would help to make the flowers grow. Mason remembered the times when Petey got out of his cage and flew around his room. They shared many memories. Mason's mother told him that the flowers would be a good way to remember Petey. Mason shared his new understanding about the cycle of life by telling his mother that Petey was helping the flowers to grow.

Although children might have more involved questions about what happens to an animal's body when it is buried in the earth, it is important to remember to keep your answers simple. Give children only as much information as they would like to know. Mason was satisfied with his mother's answer. However, an older child might have asked more detailed questions. Just as in answering questions about conception and birth, too much information can be confusing to a child. By allowing children to lead in asking what they need to know, you are able to appropriately assist them in gathering information to work through the loss.

Multiple Losses

For children coping with multiple losses, the need for denial might be greater and can pose significant challenges for the therapist. The therapist needs to distinguish between the losses and bring the remote losses to the surface, then remove them one by one, starting with the most recent loss the child is experiencing. An example of such a situation is a child who experienced the death of her grandmother, then a few months later experienced the deaths of her grandfather and her pet hamster. Another example is a child who lost both of his parents and the family dog in a car accident.

Janelle

Janelle, age 14 years, experienced the death of her 19-year-old brother Leroy (who died from an unexpected coronary incident), her cat, and then her dog within a 2-week period. The loss of her brother severely taxed the family's emotional, financial, and spiritual resources and delayed a grief response for the loss of animals. Although the parents grieved the loss of their son, they were not able to cope with saying good-bye to the family pets. The grief they felt was a tidal wave of emotion in response to tragedy hitting the daughter and both parents not once but three times. This family sought professional support. Janelle and her parents had to come to terms with the loss of Leroy before addressing the additional loss of two family pets. After working through much of her immediate grief, Janelle shared with the therapist her belief that her dog and cat went to join Leroy in heaven. She said that it gave her comfort to imagine that all three of them were together and that Leroy was not alone.

Compound Loss

Although multiple losses can occur simultaneously or close together, compound loss can occur over many years. Children can be reminded (either while awake or in dreams) of other losses from the past. Although the majority of pet losses might be a child's first loss and experience with feelings of grief and death, some children do experience a number of losses throughout their childhoods. These losses can include the loss of other pets and people, moves, and changes in family structure (as I mentioned previously). Children who are in foster care are at a higher risk for experiencing compound loss. The compounded effect of past, present, and anticipated loss can be overpowering. A full and accurate assessment of past losses experienced by the child needs to be made. How the child coped with past losses needs to be documented as well. A child experiencing compound loss might be experiencing multiple losses at once or might be recalling unresolved losses from the past.

The therapist's job is to help the client sort through previous losses, validating them and identifying coping strengths that the child displayed at the time of the loss. Unresolved losses from the past can be identified, and effective coping strategies used to resolve past grief and loss can be used again. Most likely, though, the child will need support in gaining new coping strategies and using them in working through the current and unresolved losses.

Bargaining

Children will often bargain in an attempt to feel as if they have some control over the outcome of their pet's fate. Children might bargain for their pet to return. They might bargain with God or with their parents or with the veterinarian to make their pet well, and they might promise to be good and do their homework or to be nice to their siblings in an attempt to change the pet's fate. Children might attempt to do what they promise in the hope that the pet will be found alive or come back to life. When bargaining fails, the denial dissipates and the child progress through the grief process. However, not all children will bargain. They might move from the initial phase of shock to another phase.

Anger

Anger surfaces when denial breaks down and the child realizes that no amount of bargaining will bring the pet back. It is not uncommon for a child to yell at the parents, "I hate you!" or to accuse the veterinarian of killing the pet. In most cases, this anger is short-lived and dissipates once the child has had time to assimilate all the facts related to the pet's illness or death. When the anger is projected outward, it can remain there in a sort of holding pattern that actually protects the child from the impact of his or her own rage.

I watched as a veterinarian approached a family to tell them that their dog had died, and the young child responded to the news by slamming an exam room door in the veterinarian's face. If the child feels guilty of some neglect or feels responsible in some way for the demise of the pet, that knowledge can break through the child's defenses and the child might turn the anger on himself or herself. Typically, guilt lies at the root of the rage and anger a child is feeling. As with any child in crisis, the therapist must remain alert for danger signals that might warrant a further evaluation of the child in a safer environment. Maintaining a calm presence when emotions of rage, anger, and fear are being expressed will help to calm the child. The anger can give way to tears, expressions of remorse, and fear of abandonment. The child needs not only to be told but also to feel that he or she is not going to be abandoned and that you are there to help. Acknowledging the child's feelings and validating the depth of the loss are the first steps in helping a child who is coping with a myriad emotions.

Guilt

Most people who experience the loss of a pet report feelings of guilt. This is no different for children. If present in the child, guilt poses the greatest obstacle to the child's resolving the loss. It is important to alleviate guilt feelings as early as possible (see chapter 4, "Special Types of Loss," the case example about Erica and Mickey). Children often tend to blame themselves even without have any real reason to do so. They wonder if the pet died because of something they did or did not do. Their beliefs can be based on real or imagined omissions or errors. The child might express feelings of guilt out loud or might express them in a drawing, as did the very young boy whose mother told him that his pet hamster died because he had forgotten to feed it (mentioned in a previous chapter).

Uncovering guilty feelings might involve more creative endeavors by the therapist. Feelings that the child is resistant to share can be written down and placed in a "secrets" jar for the therapist to read. The child might express guilt through play or storytelling. The objective of therapy should be to enable the child to express the guilt and then carefully explore it with the therapist. Children experiencing guilt must be reminded that they did all that they could within their physical, emotional, and cognitive abilities. In the example of the young child who forgot to feed his pet, the therapist should remind the child (and the parents) that young children do not have the ability to predict the consequences of their actions or inactions. Statements made to children out of anger or frustration and without thought can be damaging and have lasting effects. A comment a caregiver makes to a child regarding the injury or death of a pet might be long forgotten by the caregiver when the child begins to exhibit emotional difficulties. It is the therapist's job to assist the child in uncovering the source of the guilt feelings. Once identified, the therapist and child are able to work through the guilt issues. One way to assist a child who is experiencing guilt is to reframe the event for the child.

Reframing

While acknowledging the child's role in the pet's death, the therapist reframes the event to include all of the facts and demonstrates that the child made the best possible choice given the situation and information available to him or her.

Understanding what it is the child is expressing is paramount to helping the child through the loss. An effective way to work with a child who is having difficulty expressing the loss is to have the child tell the story of the experience. The therapist draws a detailed picture of the child's story. The therapist then presents the picture to the child, asking, "I think this picture explains how you're feeling. Am I right?" If the child says no, the therapist asks the child to make corrections or to draw a picture of his or her own. This works best with young children. The therapist needs to take an imaginary snapshot of the child's emotional experience with loss and present it (often verbally) to the child for validation. Once the impact of the loss is fully identified, the therapist will be able to reframe the experience for the child in a way that is conducive to healing. When a child experiences grief, an authoritarian approach is best avoided. Gentle and repeated questioning and reframing of the events will be necessary to help the child establish a healthier perception of the event.

The following story is an example of reframing. Julia, a 7-year-old, stated to the therapist, "I killed Emma." The therapist replied, "You are saying that you killed your bunny, Emma." Julia: "Uh huh. I left her in the sun and she died." Therapist: "You left Emma in the sun and she became overheated and then died." Julia: "Yup." Therapist: "Your mom told me that you were cleaning the area around Emma's cage and she asked you to move her out of the way." Julia: "I moved her into the place that wasn't sunny." Therapist: "While you and your mom were cleaning, the sun changed position and shined on Emma. She became overheated in the sun and died. You put her there because your mom told you to move the cage. You and your mom didn't know that sun would change position and that too much sun could cause Emma to die." Julia, quietly: "No." Therapist: "You loved Emma and took very good care of her. You wouldn't do something that would hurt her." Julia: "No, but I did." Therapist: "It was an accident, something that you didn't expect or want to happen. Accidents sometimes happen to people and animals. When they do, people need to forgive themselves and each other. You didn't put Emma in the sun on purpose or expect her to die." Julia: "No, I loved Emma."

While acknowledging the child's role in the pet's death, the therapist reframes the event to include all of the facts and demonstrates that the child made the best possible choice given the situation and information available to her. The reframing allows the child to see herself as a loving and caring pet owner who made a mistake for which she should not harbor guilt feelings.

Prolonged Despair

A loss of all hope that things will get better or that the child will feel good again is not part of the normal grieving process when it continues for a significant period of time (2 weeks or longer). Children who feel this way are stuck in the grieving process, and the therapist needs to discover an effective method to move them quickly through this phase.

A child who has a weak or absent support system might have regarded the pet as the only one who truly cared for him or her. The child might feel intense loneliness, and his or her will to participate in normal activities can be seriously diminished. In addition, guilt associated with the death of the pet can damage a child's self-esteem so much that he or she can disengage from social activities, refusing to go to school, take care of personal hygiene, eat, play with other children, or get up in the morning. A child who is feeling this way should be assessed for clinical depression.

Substance Abuse

In our society, children can see and hear that alcohol and drugs will make a hurt go away. Caregivers can unwittingly state in front of children that they need a drink because they had a hard day. In the popular cartoon *Zits,* the father is frustrated with his teenage son Jeremy's inability to take phone messages, and he tells the mother to bring him a chardonnay. In movies and on television, children can witness characters' numbing their pain by taking a drink, and "I need a drink" is a statement children often hear. Children might mimic these behaviors by turning to alcohol and drugs in an attempt to self-medicate or to escape intense feelings of hopelessness, guilt, loneliness, and despair. Alcohol use will only temporarily serve to make the person feel better by dulling pain. Children need to be told that alcohol should not be used to avoid pain because it can make them ill or because too much could kill them. They need to be informed of the fact that although there are pharmaceutical medicines available to help people feel better, these need to be prescribed by a physician and are different from street drugs that are sold as something to make you feel great. Children need to be told that drugs offered to them on the street could harm or kill them. Children who are using need to have immediate interventions and be helped with appropriate substance-abuse programs while being helped through their grief.

Suicide

The loss of a pet can sometimes evoke suicidal thoughts in children, especially in those who do not have a good support system. Children are at a higher risk for suicide if someone in their immediate family has committed suicide. Any suicidal gestures in children should be taken seriously. Children are not always forthcoming about their feelings. Very young children who do not understand or possess enough language to express their level of despair can express their feelings in other ways. Children can write their feelings down, and they can draw a picture of how they feel, which they might show to a friend, parent, teacher, or some other trusted person. Children who are told by another child that he or she wants to commit suicide should tell a trusted adult immediately. Most children who have taken their lives have informed at least one other person prior to making the attempt. Some adults might view the child's threat of suicide as being overly dramatic. Any and all comments need to be taken seriously and not considered to be manipulative or acting out on the part of the child.

Children might say it casually or they might scream out the fact that they want to end their lives. They might view suicide as a way of ending the pain they feel over the death of the pet that died. They might wish to die to relieve guilt feelings, and they might have depressing thoughts over a loss and want to join their pet that died. They might think suicidal thoughts and be afraid to share them. Their behavior might change, and they might withdraw or act out. Children might join in dangerous dare games such as attempting to jump out a window or driving dangerously. They might say they hate themselves and do things to hurt themselves, like cutting their arms. Some talk about music they would like to have played at their funerals. Children, even very young children, do attempt suicide, and some succeed. Children who are feeling this way need immediate intervention by a skilled therapist. Children need to feel that life is worth living and that they can get help to work through their losses and accompanying feelings.

If a caregiver has reason to suspect that a child is thinking of suicide, the following steps should be taken:

1. Ask the child if he or she is planning on committing suicide.
2. If the answer is yes, inquire if the child has a plan in place.
3. Ask what means the child will use.

Immediately get the child to a safe place where a full psychiatric evaluation can be made and the child can be helped. Let the child know that you will not give up on him or her and that you will stay with him or her; then do it.

Lisa and Brinley

Lisa, a ninth grader in high school, experienced the sudden and unexpected death of her German shepherd Brinley when the dog was hit and killed by a car near her home. Lisa told several of her friends about her loss. Many said that they were sorry. In the weeks that followed, Lisa's behavior changed. She would sit by herself under a tree on the front lawn of the school during lunchtime with her sweatshirt pulled over her head. When her friends tried to engage her in lunch or other activities, she told them to leave her alone. She shared with one of her closest friends, Lauren, that she planned to kill herself. Lauren had known Lisa to be overly dramatic and to say and do what Lauren referred to as "stupid stuff" in the past. However, she was concerned enough to share this information with her mother. Her mother asked Lauren if she could call Lisa's mother. Lauren refused and said it would be a betrayal of her friendship because Lisa had made Lauren promise not to tell. Lauren's mother assured her that Lisa's comment about committing suicide was a cry for help and that they needed to tell someone who could help Lisa right away. She explained to Lauren that Lisa might actually kill herself or attempt to do so and hurt herself, and as Lisa's friends they needed to help Lisa. Lauren agreed to let her mother tell the school counselor on the condition that she remained anonymous. Lauren's mother agreed and promptly contacted Lisa's school counselor.

Lisa was removed from class and taken to the counseling office. There she met with her counselor and her parents. Lisa was taken for a psychiatric evaluation. She said that she was depressed over the loss of her dog and wanted to die but did not have a plan for doing so. The decision was made to place Lisa in therapy, along with her family, and start her on antidepressants.

Several weeks later, Lisa contacted Lauren. Lisa told Lauren that she was calling to thank her. Lisa credited Lauren with saving her life. Lisa said to Lauren that she was pretty messed up after Brinley died and because of some other things going on in her life. Lauren asked Lisa why she thought it was Lauren who had told. Lisa said she did not have proof, but she trusted Lauren and thought that Lauren might have told someone who could help her.

Although Lauren's mother was placed in an awkward position—not wanting to betray her daughter's trust but at the same time wanting to help her daughter's friend—she helped both girls by educating Lauren about suicide and by reporting Lisa's statement to someone who was in a position to intervene. The school responded by taking Lisa's statement seriously and immediately talking to her about it. Lisa was able to get the support of her school, her family, the medical community, and her friend during a time when she was in crisis.

Conclusion

Although most children will successfully work through a loss and find the support they need to continue to integrate the experience into their lives, sometimes the loss of a pet can trigger unusual, intense responses in children. Normal grief responses, carried to the extreme, might require crisis intervention. In these cases, children will need more support and therapeutic interventions. The loss of a companion animal can be as intense and painful for the child as the loss of a human family member or friend. As such, the loss must be acknowledged and validated before any intervention can succeed. Children need to be educated about and assessed for alcohol and drug abuse. Children who are using are at a greater risk of harming themselves or dying.

Children can and do commit suicide. Any overtures, statements, gestures, writings, or drawings indicating that the child is considering ending his or her life should be taken seriously, and the child should be promptly helped.

8

TYPES OF SUPPORT AND
THERAPIES FOR CHILDREN

Friendship doubles our joys and halves our grief.
—Dolley Madison

The grief experience can be so overwhelming for a family that sometimes children are overlooked. Parents can be so enveloped in their own feelings of loss and despair that they neglect to assist their children with their feelings. Furthermore, children are not always able to articulate their feelings coherently or directly.

Therapists and other caregivers can provide children with a confidant, someone to trust with whom they can share their deepest, even secret, feelings. Sharing grief helps children who feel they are carrying the burden of the loss alone. It also allows children to help each other during a difficult time in which they might feel lost, alone, angry, scared, sad, and guilty. One of the most effective ways to receive and give support is in a group setting, one run by a therapist skilled in helping children. In a pet loss group, meeting other children who have experienced the loss of a pet helps children to know that they are not alone in their grief. In a pet loss support group, friendships are born and validation for heartfelt emotions is expressed. Although group settings are ideal for older children, a group setting that includes play therapy might be better suited to younger children.

In this chapter I discuss the types of therapies caregivers can use in assisting children through the loss of a pet. I include a brief overview with a description of the therapy and examples of how it has been effectively used to assist children. More in-depth discussions on the therapeutic benefits of therapies for children dealing with compound loss and other complications that can hinder the grieving process can be found in chapter 7.

Cognitive Therapy

Cognitive therapy is one of the therapies a professional can use in assisting a child through a loss. Cognitive therapy relies on learning principles that involve cognition (perception, thinking, reasoning, attention, and judgment). The strategy is to change the thoughts, beliefs, assumptions, and attitudes that contribute to the child's emotional or behavioral problems. The cognitive therapy approach assumes that children who are experiencing depression view themselves negatively and that this type of thinking is distorted. They might exhibit an "all or none" type of thinking or look at all events and actions as "good or bad," with nothing in the middle. A therapist will assist a child in first recognizing this behavior and then changing it. I include a case example using cognitive therapy in this chapter.

Behavioral Therapy

Behavioral therapy is used to eliminate or reduce unwanted reactions to bodily sensations or functions, which includes exposure therapy (showing the child a picture of what is feared and eventually allowing the child to experience the feared situation), contingency management (rewarding desirable actions and ignoring undesirable actions), behavioral activation (developing a list of activities the child used to enjoy and obtaining the child's agreement to carry them out), modeling (having the child observe other children in the situation that is feared and see that nothing harmful or negative results from the experience), and biofeedback (using instrumentation to help learn to control bodily activities, such as muscle tension). Many therapists find that they have the most success in combining cognitive and behavioral therapy techniques in working with clients.

Art Therapy

Art therapy uses paint, pens, charcoal, clay, and other media to allow children to create images through which to explore feelings, dreams, memories, and ideas. Children experiencing a pet loss can find relief, strengthen insight, and find courage to explore feelings in depth through art therapy. Creativity can provide a means of expression for that which is difficult to express in words or is not fully understood. The art therapist uses the child's art as a point of reference in helping the child to further explore feelings, perceptions, and experiences and find clarity and meaning in his or her life.

Art therapy can be used to assist a child of almost any age. Very young children do not have the verbal capacity to fully express everything they are feeling about a loss. A child might be better able to draw or paint feelings than to attach words to their emotions. One 8-year-old child who lost his dog drew a picture of himself feeling sad. He then drew another picture beside it of him feeling happy. He wrote captions above both his sad and happy selves. The caption above the sad self read, "My dog died." The caption above his happy self read, "Maybe I will get another dog." This child was able to demonstrate that he felt deep feelings of loss about the death of his dog, and he was also able to express that he expected to feel happiness in having another dog to bond with someday. Another child drew a picture of her cat. The cat was very beautiful in the picture. She then drew a picture of a road behind the cat. "This is where my cat was killed, on the road," she sadly explained when describing her picture. Another child, a 7-year-old boy, drew a picture of his hamster living in a cage. He drew a food dish filled with food, a water bottle filled with water, and an exercise wheel. He also drew the hamster. When asked to talk the picture, he was careful to talk about the water bottle, food dish, and wheel. He said that one morning he found his hamster dead in the cage. When the therapist commented on the water in the bottle, the food in the dish, and the exercise wheel, noting that the hamster in the picture was well cared for, the boy said that he might have not cared for his hamster that well. He explained that his mother told him that the hamster might have died because he forgot to feed his hamster. The boy then tried to remember at what time of day he fed his hamster and if indeed there had been days when he had forgotten. He was clearly distressed at having learned that he might have been responsible for the demise of his pet.

The insight and knowledge a therapist can gain from a picture or image produced by a child can significantly enhance the therapeutic process of working through a loss. A child might not be able to articulate guilt but be able to draw the images representing feelings of guilt and then find a way to organize and articulate his or her thoughts. Also, beliefs about death and loss can be revealed when the child describes a drawing; for example, "When I see the road where my cat was killed I feel sad. When I think of her in heaven I'm happy because I know she is looking down on me." These are significant insights into a child's belief system on which a therapist can build when working with a child.

Art therapy can be applied almost anywhere, any time. Many times at the support group, children draw pictures that they might or might not want to share with the group. Through the picture they are able to tell the stories about what happened to their pets and how they feel about it.

Play Therapy

Play therapy can be extremely useful in assisting a young child through grief and loss. In her book *Play Therapy,* Virginia Axline summed up the play therapy experience for a very young boy who was facing a second surgery on his throat.

The child worked through his anticipatory anxiety about the procedure while playing with finger paints in the playroom. Holding up his hands covered in red paint, the boy stated, "Sometimes it bleeds! Look! Bloody like my throat." Axline wrote, "As he pins his thoughts and feelings down on paper he feels, perhaps, more secure. After he has captured them on paper he can handle them a little better. This is his fear and his anxiety. Now he can see it—touch it—feel it. He is no longer at the mercy of some nameless fear he can control in this manner."[1]

Axline discussed the importance of accepting the child completely during a play therapy session so he can achieve the courage to express his true feelings. The therapist does not praise the child for actions performed, nor does the therapist's acceptance imply approval. What the therapist does during play therapy is accurately reflect back what the child is expressing. Axline stated, "Play therapy offers children an opportunity to work through their problems, to learn and to know themselves, to accept themselves as they are, and to grow more mature through the therapy experience."[2] The child is the one directing the play, choosing the things that are important to him, assuming the responsibility for making the decisions in the playroom. He does the interpreting and the working through of his problems in a place in which he feels safe. Through the process, the child will gain respect for himself as a person of value.

During play therapy, children can act out their feelings and problems. Play therapy is an opportunity for children to work through a grief experience and the accompanying feelings. Ultimately children can alleviate their fears and anxieties through play therapy.

Jane Annunziata, Psy.D. in clinical psychology from Rutgers University and coauthor of *A Child's First Book About Play Therapy* stated,

> Psychoanalytic play therapy is based on an assumption that children's problems stem from unconscious conflicts and developmental deficits that will reveal themselves in their play. Through their play, their verbalizations, and their relationship to the therapist, children can be helped to understand what is troubling them. A child's behavior (problematic or not) is taken to be an attempt at meaningful communication of underlying thoughts and feelings, and, through therapeutic understanding of the child's communications, resolution of problem behaviors can occur.[3]

She continued, "Psychoanalytic play therapy includes the involvement of the child's parents. The therapist's familiarity with the child's parents helps the child feel accurately understood (which facilitates the resolution of the child's difficulties)." Furthermore, this involvement provides parents with practical strategies for managing problematic behaviors at home. Symptoms can then improve and troublesome behaviors diminish in frequency and intensity. In addition to working with parents, child therapists often coordinate with schoolteachers and counselors to help resolve any behavioral difficulties at school and increase understanding of the child's emotional issues.

> In psychoanalytic play therapy, the child takes the lead in producing 'material' in the form of play. It is a nondirective approach in which the therapist follows the child and not vice versa. When the therapist is careful to avoid giving advice or making suggestions, the child becomes increasingly able to reveal his or her emotional life in spontaneous play. The therapist attempts to understand what the child is communicating through his or her play (i.e., what the child is thinking and

feeling, both consciously and unconsciously). As the child plays, the therapist comments on the play itself, its underlying (latent) meaning, and its relation to presenting symptomatology.[4]

Therapists will be most effective with children without being overly solicitous or condescending if the children can be themselves, willing to play at ease. The therapist should create a comfortable environment in which children are able to express their concerns through play.

Who Can Benefit From Play Therapy?

Annunziata suggested that play therapy is recommended for children between the ages of 3 and 11 years who present a wide variety of emotionally based difficulties. These include children who have problems relating to peers, problems with appropriate expression of anger, childhood depression, anxiety, adjustment reactions to specific life events, school difficulties that have an emotional component, deficits in self-esteem, and withdrawal. Other difficulties include more severe character pathology, attention-deficit disorders, development disorders, and symptoms inappropriate to the youngster's current age (such as enuresis and encopresis). When a child experiences any of these difficulties to such an extent that symptoms are pronounced, recurrent, or continual, treatment might be indicated.

The following factors are considered when determining whether treatment is indicated:

- how long the problem has persisted
- if the problem is interfering with family life
- if the child is experiencing significant internal distress, even though overt symptoms might be subtle
- if attempts have been made in the past to help the child overcome the problem
- how disruptive the problem is to the child's daily functioning

- if the problem is interfering with academic performance
- if the problem is interfering with normal maturation
- if the problem is unusual for the child's developmental stage
- if the problem is actually embedded in a pattern of symptoms[5]

Eva and Tulip

Eva was a bright, outgoing, 8-year-old girl who lived at home with her parents, a dog named Alexia, and her two older brothers. Recently the family had experienced the loss of their English bulldog Tulip. Tulip had lived with Eva her entire life. After the death of Tulip, Eva argued frequently with her brothers, cried easily, and was short tempered with her family. Her brothers, ages 12 and 14, although not reported by their parents to be abusive in their behavior toward their sister, did engage in a fair amount of sibling rivalry that included teasing Eva.

During the first play therapy session, Eva chose to play with a dollhouse. She included a mother doll, sister doll, two brother dolls, and two small toy dogs in her play. Eva played quietly while the therapist observed her. Eva spoke very quietly as she moved the figures around the house. The therapist commented, "Eva, you are speaking very softly." Eva replied, "Yes. I just want to play by myself." The therapist said, "Yes, you want to play with the dollhouse by yourself." Eva continued to play as the therapist continued to observe quietly. After a few more minutes, Eva closed the doors of the dollhouse and then further explored the playroom. Eva walked over to the puppets and commented that there were many puppet animals, including a monkey, a bird, a cat, and a dog. The therapist said, "We have many animal puppets." Eva then asked the therapist if she would like to see what was inside the dollhouse. The therapist said, "You want me to come see what is inside the dollhouse?" Eva opened the doors. The therapist saw that one of the brother dolls was lying face up on the floor in one of the bedrooms. One of the toy dogs stood on the brother doll's head, while the other dog was positioned on top of the brother doll's legs, pinning him to the floor while the sister doll was standing nearby. The therapist described to Eva what she saw. Eva told her that the dogs were protecting the sister doll from the mean brother. "The dog protects the sister from the brother," the therapist said to Eva.

After two more play sessions, the therapist learned that Eva's dogs had protected her from her brothers when they were being mean. The meanness was reported by Eva to include teasing her, chasing her, yelling at her, and slamming doors on her. Eva said that she loved and missed Tulip and that she now only had Alexia to protect her. The dogs, she said, made her feel safe. Many of these incidents in which Eva described not feeling safe had taken place when her parents were not at home. After the therapist talked to Eva's mother, she and Eva's father decided to meet with the family and to address the behavior that was taking place, primarily when they were not at home, and the consequences that would be enforced if the behavior continued. They also hired a babysitter for Eva when they had to leave her unattended. Eva agreed to this arrangement. During the fifth and final play session, Eva's mother reported that there was less fighting in the house (although a significant amount of sibling rivalry still existed). Eva appeared to be happier and easier going. The mother also reported that her oldest son had expressed his relief at having a sitter look after Eva, as she usually refused to listen to him when the parents were not at home.

Family Therapy

Family therapy is another way in which children can work through feelings associated with a pet loss while being supported by the family and addressing all of the family's concerns about the loss. Many times families seek out support

when they have experienced the loss of a pet or are considering euthanizing a pet or allowing it to be adopted into another
home. Complicating factors can be divorce, a move, a loss of
a therapeutic animal (e.g., a seeing-eye dog), drug and alcohol abuse, a death of a human family member, multiple losses,
and other physical and psychological issues present at the
time of loss.

Our families can influence our perceptions, our modes of
interacting, and our styles of communicating. In family
therapy, the therapist applies therapeutic principles while
engaging the participation of family members, individually
and as a group. The process recognizes and reinforces con-
structive aspects of the family's relationships while also allowing destructive elements and counterproductive interaction
styles to be identified, acknowledged, and changed. Although
the idea of family is usually understood in the traditional
sense as a mother, father, and children, a family is considered to be any group of individuals who are committed to
one another's well-being.

The following case study is about a family that witnessed
the traumatic loss of their dog as it was run over by a speed-
ing truck in front of their home.

The Miller Family

Daughter Angie, 11 years old, and son Peter, 9 years old, witnessed their dog being run over by a truck in front of their
house while they were playing on the front lawn. The parents, Mike and Sharon, brought their children to therapy to
help them work through their feelings regarding the loss.

The family wept openly for their German shepherd Tuffy
and talked about how empty their home seemed without him.
The children had witnessed the dog's running out into the
street (through a gate that was left open by Angie) and the
truck's hitting him. They expressed their anger that the truck
driver had not stopped to help Tuffy. They all spoke about
the blood-soaked asphalt in front of their house. The father

reported weeping each time he drove into the driveway, and the mother described her repeated attempts at washing the spot from the asphalt. They admitted to a lot of tension in the household with the children and parents frequently arguing and tempers easily flaring.

The family worked hard on their grief issues in therapy. They finally made the decision to move from their home. Prior to making this rather drastic decision, they had to work through their negative feelings and forgive one another for their roles in this loss. The issues surrounding the loss involved Peter's anger toward Angie for leaving the gate open, which allowed the dog to run out of the yard and into the street. This also included the parents' harboring resentment toward Angie, too, although their resentment was veiled by their genuine attempts to be supportive of their daughter at the same time. There were also conflicts between the parents about their inability to help their children through this traumatic experience.

Peter and Angie were reported to have been experiencing nightmares, fatigue, tearfulness, and short tempers with each other. Both children were seen separately for eye movement reprocessing therapy (discussed in depth later in this chapter) to eliminate the persistent images of the pet's death. After the first two sessions, the parents reported a positive change in the children's demeanors. The children seemed to be sleeping solidly, and the nightmares and persistent thoughts seemed to have diminished.

Therapy sessions also included just the parents together, the children together, and several whole family sessions. During the family sessions, the therapist helped them to see that the incident was the result of an unintentional mistake made by a child. The therapist guided them toward forgiveness of one another for the roles they played in the loss. Sharon forgave Mike for being crabby and distant. She forgave Peter for being difficult and for fighting with his sister. She forgave Angie for making a mistake, one that could have been made by any member of the family. Finally, she forgave herself for harboring resentment toward her daughter and for arguing with her husband. Each family member took a turn in the process of forgiveness to attain closure. The Millers made a decision, as a family, to move from their home, as they did not want to continue to see the spot where Tuffy was killed.

Although this seems like an extreme measure, for this family it had therapeutic value. Their attempts to "wash away" the memory of the accident had failed. The spot remained, even though they were able to work through their feelings of loss, anger, and guilt. They believed that a physical move from the site would spare them from the ever-present reminder. The therapist supported that decision.

Storytelling

Storytelling is another effective way to work with young children. Children are able to identify feelings and safely discuss them in a nondirective, nonthreatening way. Children can make up stories about feelings, using their own metaphors to express heartfelt emotions in a made-up or fantasy way. There are several books for children about feelings associated with animals and death (see chapter 10). In many of these books, children are encouraged to make up stories about their pets. This activity allows them to mix fantasy and reality and helps them to safely and effectively work through their feelings. In Barbara Kay Polland's book *Feelings: Inside You and Outloud Too,* children can choose any photo and make up a story about it.[6]

The following case example illustrates how the use of storytelling assisted a young boy in expressing how the loss of the family dog, and the subsequent parents' fighting as a result of not working through their grief issues, was affecting him.

Kyle

Six-year-old Kyle's father and mother frequently argued about the loss of their 9-year-old Irish setter. Apparently in response to these arguments, Kyle often cried and refused to play with his friends. He also told his parents how much he loved them and tried to hug them when they were in the middle of an argument.

Kyle's parents became concerned when his teacher noted this type of behavior at school. The parents decided to consult a therapist who worked with children. Kyle was told that he was going to see a "worry doctor," someone who helps with worries. The therapist asked Kyle to look at the book of photos titled *Feelings: Inside You and Outloud Too.* She told Kyle he could choose any photo in the book and make up a story about it.

Kyle chose a picture of a man walking down the front steps of a house. A little boy sat in the window with a sad expression on his face, watching the man. Kyle said the man was the boy's father, and that the father was mad and was leaving his son because their dog had died.

The therapist determined that Kyle thought his parents were angry with him and might leave because of the loss of their dog. Kyle's parents reassured him that they were not going to leave him, that they were not angry with him, and that they did not blame him for the death of their dog. They apologized for arguing in front of him and told him that, despite their angry and sad feelings regarding the dog's death, they still loved each other and were committed to working through the loss as a family. The family then worked together on acceptable solutions for managing the anger stage of the grieving process.[7]

Trauma Work

Assisting a child through a traumatic loss takes knowledge, skill, patience, and creativity. Because children are continu-

ing to develop cognitively, a child who experiences a traumatic pet loss at age 5 years will continue to process the
experience and work on the loss as he or she grows and gains
more knowledge. Open communication and willingness by
the caregiver to provide the child with the support needed to
fully work through a loss is key in helping to ensure good
mental health in the child. It is not uncommon for a child to
question a loss, especially a traumatic one, a year or more
after it occurred. Children should not be told to forget about
it or to put it out of their minds. They need support in working through all the issues that arise with the loss, especially
if those issues arise long after the loss occurred. If children
feel safe in asking questions and expressing their feelings,
they will have more opportunity to work through those feelings and ultimately resolve the loss. Children can become
stuck in the grieving process when they are not encouraged
to explore their feelings to the fullest.

Although there are a variety of therapeutic ways in which
to assist children through traumatic losses (described previously), there is a newer therapy that can be used in conjunction with other therapies and has been reported to be highly
effective in children and adults.

On a daily basis, we all use our minds to figure things out,
cope with predictable stresses, and regulate our emotions
and our self-esteem. But the experience of trauma can overwhelm our capacity to cope, and the trauma experience often
gets stored in our minds in ways that make it difficult to use
our usual ways of coping. Of particular challenge to a therapist is the child who witnessed the traumatic death of a pet.
A therapy that can be particularly helpful is eye movement
desensitization and reprocessing (EMDR). This type of
therapy is widely used and assists the brain with its natural
processing of emotional information. This therapeutic intervention was developed by Francine Shapiro, Ph.D., in 1987
and can be used in conjunction with other therapies with
children and adults who have sustained trauma.

EMDR

The EMDR therapist assists the child's healing process by becoming a partner on a journey that can change the way the child feels about himself or herself. The therapist gently guides the child to pinpointing a problem emotion or event that becomes the target of treatment. For example, one child helplessly stood by as a dog killed her cat. After a couple of months, although this traumatic event was in her past, she could not think about the event without experiencing the emotions associated with the loss. She still had feelings of guilt, helplessness, anger, and grief. However, after receiving EMDR therapy from a trained and qualified therapist, she was able to remember the event without experiencing the emotions associated with it.

Typically, children who have experienced a loss can develop a negative way of thinking about themselves. They might blame themselves for the loss or feel that they are somehow bad because of it. These negative feelings affect their self-esteem and thus affect all areas of their lives, from developing friendships to performing academically and athletically. The EMDR procedure can help desensitize the images and feelings associated with the traumatic loss and thus help the child to think more positively about himself or herself in relation to the event.

How EMDR Works

The therapist talks to the child and the parent in an effort to obtain a personal history, understand the child, and determine how the difficulty is currently affecting the child's life. Once this information is obtained, the therapist and child work together to construct a description of the problem (e.g., witnessing a dog kill her cat), negative perceptions the child has about himself or herself in relation to this event (e.g., "I felt helpless," "I did nothing," "I was afraid," "I'm a bad person because I did not save my cat," "I hate that dog"), and emotions and physical sensations associated with the event. If the child is old enough, the therapist asks the child to rate numerically the degree of upset and credibility of positive beliefs so that the child's progress can be monitored.

Once this protocol is established, the therapist and child begin the processing phase of the procedure by using the eye movements (or other kinds of attentional stimulation such TheraTapper, a light bar, or recordings for auditory bilateral stimulation; more information on these can be found in chapter 10).

Although there is a variety of ways in which a therapist incorporates EMDR into therapy, a typical EMDR session lasts between 60 and 90 minutes. During this treatment, the therapist is facing the child. The therapist asks the child to bring to mind the picture of the experience that is bothering him or her and any negative self-statements, emotions, and physical sensations associated with the traumatic experience. The child is asked to hold these images in mind while watching the therapist's hand moving rapidly back and forth (or receiving any other type of bilateral stimulation by the therapist). After a series of roughly 30 to 50 eye movements (or more), the therapist asks the child to stop, let go of the image (or thought) for a second, take a deep breath, and then notice and describe what thoughts, feelings, or images arose. The therapist might ask the child to continue his or her same thoughts, feelings, or images. The therapist then performs the bilateral stimulation process again. By stimulating the left and right sides of the brain, simultaneously, the therapist enables the child to reprocess the traumatic event so it no longer impedes daily functioning. As the thoughts, images, feelings, and physical sensations become less distressing, the therapist asks the child to bring up a positive self-statement (e.g., "I did the best that I could do for my cat in that situation."). The positive self-statement combined with the EMDR helps the child to associate this new way of thinking about himself or herself with the original troubling image.

Relief from symptoms can be obtained in one to six sessions, or EMDR can be a procedure the therapist uses as part of a longer term therapy. An example might be the use of hypnotherapy combined with EMDR therapy. When a traumatic event cannot easily be recalled, hypnosis can be used to uncover the traumatic event.[8]

Kathy McBeth, M.A., at the Institute for Children and Families (Westchester, PA),[9] described EMDR therapy for children as helping the child to process the experience and trauma differently. The goals of EMDR as an intervention are the following:

- focus attention on a specific memory, thought, image, or emotion
- unravel strings of disturbing traumatic experiences, possibly providing missing details or data toward resolution
- eliminate irrational components of fears to allow other expressed or hidden affect to be processed
- reinforce more adaptive behaviors
- build positive realistic beliefs
- strengthen ego and instill inner resources to build self-esteem

McBeth cautioned, "A child's developmental age is very important to determine before working with a child. A therapist using EMDR ALWAYS meets the child where he is, developmentally! A broader goal is for the child to feel successful throughout the therapeutic process. As with all therapeutic models, a child's involvement in therapy always involves the family. Depending on the child and his circumstances, a parent is sometimes physically present during the EMDR sessions. This can provide a greater security for the child."

This intervention is nontraditional, in that very little dialogue takes place during the desensitization phase of treatment. Clients who have experienced traditional talk therapy but still feel stuck on certain issues benefit greatly from EMDR. EMDR is often used in conjunction with other therapies and has been successfully used in conjunction with play therapy, family therapy, hypnosis, cognitive behavioral therapy, and others.

Psychotherapist David Grand, Ph.D., advised that one of the most effective ways to successfully work with traumatized children is by being creative. He achieves this by gearing the EMDR therapy session to the child's cognitive and developmental age and incorporates a variety of therapeutic strategies that include play, storytelling, and art. Some examples of creativity include tapping left-right-left-right on a child's shoulders, while the child draws on piece of paper (e.g., the child draws a picture of his dead fish floating in a tank). Grand uses a puppet to help very young children track right to left movement as they are telling a story. As feelings of sadness, anger, fear, and other emotions become present, Grand asks the children where they are experiencing these feelings in their bodies. Children might point to the places on their bodies or tell the therapist where they feel these feelings in their bodies, which assists children in becoming cognizant of the deeper feelings they have regarding the trauma. In addition, by having the child focus on the area in which the emotions are physically being experienced, the therapist is able to effectively incorporate the bilateral stimulation that allows the child to start processing the trauma and release it from his or her body.

I include here several case examples of treating traumatized children throughout the world. In one case example, a little girl had experienced the death of her pet cat and a year later was in a hurricane. Ricky Greenwald, in his paper titled "Applying Eye Movement Desensitization and Reprocessing (EMDR) to the Treatment of Traumatized Children: Five Case Studies," wrote,

Hurricane Andrew devastated much of South Dade County in Florida. Almost four months later, many area children were still suffering the psychological consequences, generally related to prolonged fear during the event, and subsequent loss experiences. Five such children between the ages of 4 and 11 were treated with one or two sessions of EMDR. The mother was interviewed prior to the first session and asked to describe and rate the changes in her child since the hurricane, and to respond similarly at one-week and four-week follow-up telephone interviews. All treatment and assessment was conducted by the author.[10]

Assessment measures included a structured interview in which the child's mother completed an interview covering living situation, family structure, and child's trauma history before the hurricane. The investigator used a problem rating scale and asked the mother to describe and then rate current symptoms and complaints, from 10 (*the worst the problem could be*) to 0 (*no problem at all*). The Subjective Units of Disturbance Scale (SUDS) was used during the treatment process. Treatment was continued until the parent rated the problem on the scale at 0 and there was no reactivity to the trauma endured by the child.[11]

I chose the following two examples from Greenwald because one example includes the significant loss of a family pet and the other example clearly illustrates the hidden grief and feelings that the child was unable to articulate and work through prior to EMDR treatment.

Jamie

Jamie was a precocious 4-year-old who had shown increased obstinance, clinging, and whining since the hurricane 4 months before. The first session included a complete EMDR treatment for Jamie's night fears and upsetting hurricane-related memories. The death of a cat 1 year earlier was touched on but perhaps not fully addressed. Jamie came back for a second session, mainly because she had enjoyed the first one and because she was along for the ride when her brother also returned. The second session was short and touched briefly on many items, including the death of the cat. At 1-week follow-up, her mother reported that her symptoms were back down to prehurricane levels and that she was more able to play contentedly by herself than ever before. At 4-week follow-up, her mother reported that Jamie was still sleeping alone, as she had just started to do around the beginning of treatment, and that the gains were holding steady.

Andy

Andy was an intelligent 9-year-old boy who, 2 months before the hurricane, had experienced the accidental death of a disliked classmate (he was not present at the incident). Andy's mother and he agreed that the death was the primary precipitant of his symptoms, which included being very pushy and testy, having racing thoughts that interfered with his getting to sleep, having trouble concentrating, and experiencing bad moods, and that the hurricane was just a minor intensifier of those symptoms. Six months after the classmate's death, the symptoms were not much less than when they started. Jamie believed that "it was my fault" and "I'm next [to die]."

In the first session, Andy apparently got over his guilt and need for punishment and expressed full confidence in the self-generated statements "It wasn't my fault" and "I'm going to live a long life." He was too tired to complete processing of the entire memory, and ended with a SUDS (subjective units of distress) of 6, including feelings of confusion and possible helplessness. During the next several days, Andy's parents reported that he was extremely volatile but also that he began to express and articulate difficult emotions that he had always withheld before. In the second session, the death incident was processed until the SUDS reached 0. The hurricane-related events were not addressed. At 1-week follow-up, his mother reported that his symptoms were dramatically down to just higher than the trauma baseline, with a bit of volatility remaining. His ability to express himself had continued to develop, and he was more cooperative and took more responsibility with his family than he had before. At 4-week follow-up, he was back to his pretrauma baseline, and his mother said he was "doing pretty well."[12]

EMDR Combined With Play Therapy

EMDR therapy can be highly effective when combined with play therapy in working with young children who have experienced a traumatic pet loss. Although I chose to include a case example of a girl named Stella, the details of the process of the combined therapies were not available. However, I chose this example because it made the point that when working with very young children, we can guess at or surmise a precipitating event (such as a pet loss) that leads to distressed behavior, but we might not be able to pinpoint the exact cause. Still, the therapist reports that combined therapies offered Stella relief from the anxiety she had been experiencing.

Stella

Stella was only 4 years old, but her mother was worried. For about 6 months, Stella had been different. She had been biting her nails and acting nervous, hyperactive, and bossy, and she was no longer talkative with her mother. Stella was afraid of what she referred to as the "Big Bear," which made it hard for her to get to sleep. Our best guess was that her father, with whom she no longer had contact, had scared her. Stella would not say, and there was no one else to ask. We decided to try therapy.

We spent the first few sessions doing things that make parents think that nothing is happening (because they do not see any progress a this time). I used a puppet to role-play a shy little bear. Stella got to be the one to help the bear feel comfortable. Stella learned to feel safe in my room, to feel that she was in control.

Then her concerns started coming out in her play. Big Bear! What to do? (Following Stella's lead, the play, for several sessions, centered around killing Big Bear, putting him in jail, tying him up, killing him some more.) Although Stella would pursue this activity with real drive and persistence, she also was experiencing a scary time. For a couple of sessions, she insisted that her mother sit right outside the door to the therapy room. She finally made friends with Big Bear, and then forgot about him.

A few more sessions, with a little family therapy and EMDR mixed in, and we were about done. Stella was no longer anxious or biting her fingernails, she was talkative with her mother again, and she was no longer worried about Big Bear. The funny thing about doing play therapy with young children is that sometimes you never really find out what you were working on. We do not know what made her scared. But she seemed happy again, and she stayed that way at least for the next 3 months, after which I lost contact with her mother.[12]

EMDR and Cognitive Therapy

Therapy combining EMDR and cognitive therapy for children can be very effective, as the following case illustrates. The therapy addressed the child's distorted perception of self largely inferred as a result of an upsetting grief experience in the death of his pet.

Bryan and Whitney

When Bryan was 6 months old, his 8-year-old-brother Carl found a litter of three puppies. The puppies were 9 to 10 weeks old and sickly. Bryan's family took in the pups and worked together to save them. Before long their health improved, and good homes were found for two of the puppies. Bryan's family kept the third one, a female they named Whitney.

When Bryan got older, Carl frequently reminded him that the family dog was really his because he had found and rescued Whitney, and Bryan would be wise to find a pet of his own. Bryan loved Whitney but took on two of the family cats as his own.

The years passed, and Carl grew up. He did not have time for his dog any more. Whitney lived mostly outdoors, and came indoors when the weather was bad. Eventually Bryan took over more of the dog's care. Whitney began to deteriorate in health. During the summer when both Whitney and Bryan turned 13, the family called the veterinarian twice to assess for euthanasia. Both times Whitney rallied with medication and care. In the fall of that year, the dog took a turn for the worse. The family called the veterinarian, and they decided that Whitney would be euthanized at home.

Bryan and his parents were in attendance at the euthanasia. The veterinarian they usually used was not able to perform the euthanasia that day, so they called another veterinarian. He was late, unapologetic, and not at all empathetic. He quickly assigned positions for the family, with Bryan supporting Whitney's head and the others in close attendance. Without any explanation of the procedure or possible complications, the euthanasia serum was administered and Whitney died quickly. After the veterinarian pronounced her dead, the family cried. The veterinarian requested his money and left without expressing condolences.

Bryan was confused—everything had happened in fewer than 2 minutes, without comment or evident concern for him from either the veterinarian or his parents. In truth, both parents, who were experienced with pet loss, believed there would be a brief explanation from the veterinarian to the family, as had been the parents' experience in euthanizing other pets (however, Bryan had not been included in those processes, as he was a toddler at the time). The parents reported that they did not want to usurp the role of the veterinarian by making explanations that he might not approve. The result was that no one said anything, and, incredibly, the whole procedure transpired in such an efficiently cold and detached manner that all three family members were left stunned and feeling as if they had done something wrong.

As Bryan and his parents proceeded with burial, Bryan asked his parents if he did something wrong and if the veterinarian was upset with him. Bryan's parents told him that they thought the veterinarian was tired and that ending his day with a euthanasia had been a hard thing to do. Bryan said he understood. However, his parents said that later it became apparent that he did not understand because he became moody and withdrawn. When two incidents of disciplinary problems arose at school, his parents sought counseling for their son.

Bryan's parents took him to a child psychologist for an assessment. A thorough intake was done that included interviews with both parents, with Bryan separately, and with the family together. The psychologist noted that Bryan viewed himself and the world around him negatively after the euthanasia. Bryan had self-defeating habits (fighting at school, refusing to do his homework) and faulty beliefs ("The veterinarian treated me poorly because he saw that I wasn't a good pet owner to my dog."). The therapist decided to use EMDR and cognitive therapy. The EMDR therapy targeted the euthanasia event in which Bryan's feelings of anger, guilt, and shame arose. The cognitive therapy approach was used to assist him with his perception, reasoning, and judgments that arose after the event. After several sessions, Bryan was able to view himself as being a good friend to Whitney. He was able to remember all the wonderful things he had done for her throughout her life. Bryan viewed his role in the euthanasia as a loving act of kindness to his dog. He was able to move past the anger and blame he placed on himself and see the veterinarian as a person with an indifferent attitude that had nothing to do with him or his family.

Pet Loss Support Group

Throughout the years, many families have attended the pet loss support group I run. Most referrals are from veterinarians, because a local veterinary medical association sponsors the group. I have had the privilege of working with many children of varying ages. Many of the case examples throughout this book are derived from my work with families in the group. Although the group provides clients with a safe and understanding place to express their feelings, its existence also validates their reactions to pet loss. Our society tends not to give the same level of validation to feelings about pet loss as it does to feelings about other losses. Despite education and even the advent of greeting cards that acknowledge a pet's death, the depth of the bond a person shared with an animal and the grief the person felt at the loss are not always acknowledged. In a support group setting, clients discover that their losses are not unique. They are educated about the grief process and about the human–companion animal bond. They take comfort in knowing that others share similar feelings about their pets, and they learn new, effective coping skills from the experiences of other group members. This is especially true for clients who attend a group prior to the loss of their pet. Ideally, clients should be referred to a group when they first learn or suspect that their pet is dying.

Most of the time children readily share in the discussion about their losses and are open and honest in their questions and their expression of feelings. Although some adults can feel uncomfortable sharing their feelings in front of children, it has been my experience that the adults at the pet loss support group are respectful and caring when children are present at the group. The group takes on a family type of atmosphere in which everyone shares and a bond of empathy arises. It can be a very therapeutic experience when different generations of people share their experiences regarding loss. However, the support group leader should closely monitor the sessions and be willing to provide thorough explanations regarding death and dying.

Attending a pet loss support group might be a client's first step toward seeking help, which is why a competent therapist who can assess clients for various mental and behavioral disorders should lead the group. Children and their parents might experience other losses, other stresses, or even drug and substance abuse at the same time as the pet loss. Clients can benefit from a variety of therapeutic modalities. Pet loss support groups can offer clients a form of support they cannot receive in one-on-one counseling sessions.

Pet loss support groups can complement other types of therapies. If you decide to refer a client to a support group, you can continue the one-on-one relationship you have established with the client. This relationship allows clients to meet their needs in a variety of ways. Sometimes therapists who run pet loss groups work with pet owners individually as well. The goal is to find the right combination of therapy and support to assist pet owners of any age through a loss.

When families attend a pet loss group, the group leader can employ many of the same skills used in family therapy while maintaining a shared group experience. It is often beneficial for children to hear from other children and adults outside of the family who are experiencing the loss of a pet. A child who might not easily understand her mother's feelings regarding the death of a pet can gain perspective and insight when another adult woman in the group shares similar feelings. The goal of the group is to acknowledge, validate, and support one another through the grieving process in a respectful and caring manner (see chapter 3, "Children and Euthanasia," for a case example in which children are part of a pet loss support group process).

Conclusion

Therapists need to acquaint themselves about the types of therapies that are available and the combinations that will be most effective in assisting a grieving child through a loss. Children and adults need to know that they are not alone in their feelings of grief. Feelings can be safely and effectively worked through, creating a healthy foundation on which children can build when going through future losses. Because the ways in which a pet dies can be traumatic, trauma therapy can be a component in effectively assisting a child through a loss. EMDR therapy has proved to be highly effective in assisting children and adults through loss. A therapist skilled in the various combinations of therapies will be better able to assist a child through a loss.

Although grief over the loss of a pet is not unique, unfortunately it is not always taken as seriously as human losses. Because society does not take pet loss seriously, a pet loss support group can serve to acknowledge a person's loss and validate the depth of feelings associated with the loss.

9
CHILDREN'S ARTWORK AND STORIES ABOUT LOVING AND LOSING ANIMALS

He speaketh not, and yet there lies
a conversation in his eyes.
—Henry Wadsworth Longfellow

Many children have contributed to this chapter. Through their words and artwork, the children poignantly express the attachments to their pets and feelings of loss they experienced. In both play and art, children are able to relay the depth of loss and feelings of loneliness, guilt, sadness, fear, and hope in a way that they might not have the words to articulate to a therapist or caregiver. When appropriate, I added information to the drawing or story shared.

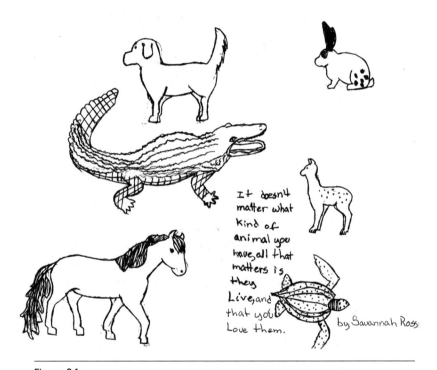

It doesn't matter what kind of animal you have, all that matters is they Live, and that you Love them.

by Savannah Rossi

Figure 9.1

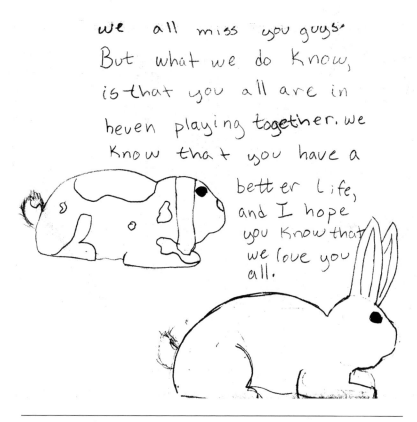

we all miss you guys. But what we do know, is that you all are in heven playing together. we know that you have a better Life, and I hope you know that we love you all.

Figure 9.2 Savannah Ross, age 11, experienced the loss of two of her rabbits, Harry and Remy, within a month of each other. Harry would often play inside the house with Savannah. She had him since she was 6 years old. As her artwork states, Savannah chose to think about Remy and Harry together in heaven. She held a funeral for Harry. Five months after his death, she was ready to bond with another rabbit, but she chose another breed.

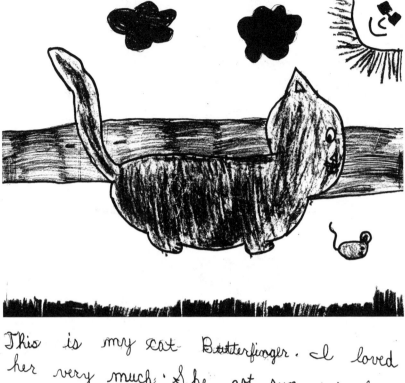

This is my cat Butterfinger. I loved her very much. She got run over by a car. When I think about her I remember that she is watching over me

by Joelle Levine age 9

Figure 9.3 Butterfinger was killed out on the road near Joelle's home. She told me that she decided to include, in her drawing, the road on which Butterfinger died. She likes to think of her cat as watching over her. Joelle experienced the death of her father and her aunt prior to losing her cat. Her father was ill for a long time. Butterfinger's death was sudden and unexpected. Joelle also became very ill after her father and aunt died. Although a healthy and happy third grader, she has endured a significant amount of loss in a short period of time. She lives at home with a loving and supportive mother and older brother.

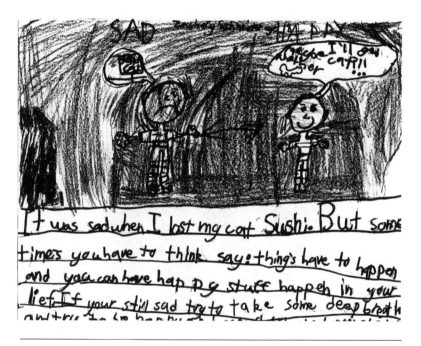

Figure 9.4

I lost my dog Wyatt when I was 4 years old. I felt sad when I lost my dog because I only had one pet in my whole life and it was taken away from me.

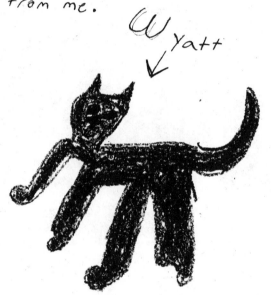

Michael Medeiros   Age 7

Figure 9.5 Michael's term "taken away from me" illustrates his unresolved feelings of anger and sadness over losing Wyatt.

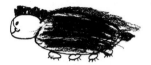

age 8¾
Jessica I.

I have a hamster named Oreo. I played with her alot and I held her alot. She was really cute, and really fun to play with. She would bite me alot. Then one day She didn't move at all. I was so afraid because when I called her name she didn't even move. When I reached to grab she was hard. She was dead. I started to cry, in fact my whole family started to cry. Even though Oreo was dead, I still dream about her every night, and I have a little hamster Beany-Baby and I pretend it's Oreo, and I play with her every day, and sometimes whenever I think of her I cry. I really loved her and I'm really sad and mad that she's gone.

Figure 9.6 It is interesting to note that Jessica included her impression of what Oreo's dead body felt like: "She was hard. She was *dead*." Pets often provide children with the opportunity to experience aspects of death that they might not encounter with people.

Age 9
Jenny Hernandez

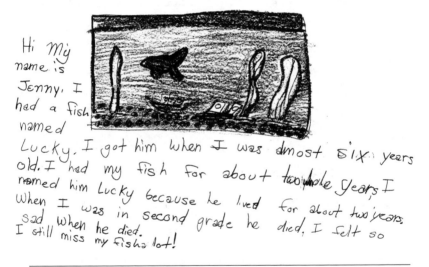

Hi my name is Jenny, I had a fish named Lucky. I got him when I was almost six years old. I had my fish for about two whole years, I named him Lucky because he lived for about two years. When I was in second grade he died, I felt so sad when he died. I still miss my fish a lot!

Figure 9.7

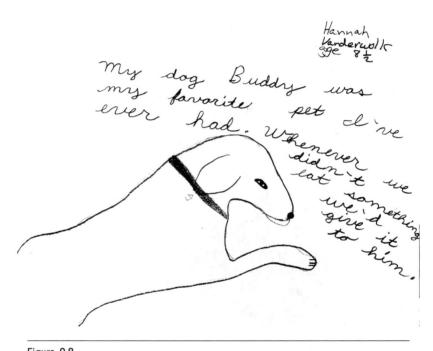

Hannah
Vanderwolk
age 8½

My dog Buddy was my favorite pet I've ever had. Whenever we didn't eat something we'd give it to him.

Figure 9.8

My dog Buck   got to live to be 14 years
old. He was very gentle and very old
for a dog. My family and I had to put
him asleep. I loved Buck and I
always will.

RyanHughes
Age8

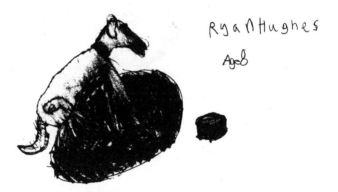

Figure 9.9

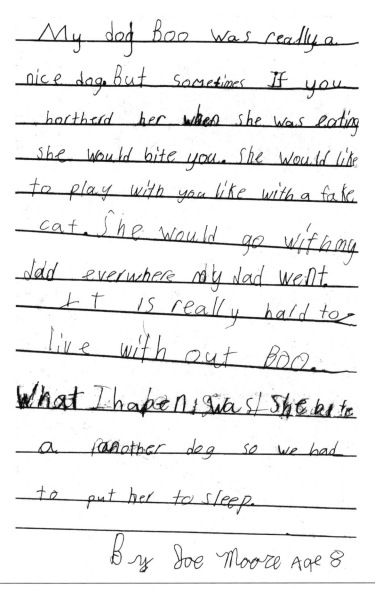

My dog Boo was really a nice dog. But sometimes If you borthered her when she was eating she would bite you. She would like to play with you like with a fake cat. She would go with my dad everwhere my dad went. It is really hard to live with out Boo. What I haben; was; she bite a fanother dog so we had to put her to sleep.

By Joe Moore Age 8

Figure 9.10

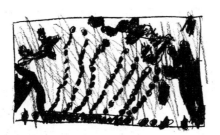

My frog's Names were Ralph and Catdog.
I had fun watching them swimming around
in a circle. I Loved feeding them when it
Was time to eat.

Freddy Peery age 10

Figure 9.11 Even the smallest of creatures can become cherished pets as poignantly illustrated by Freddy.

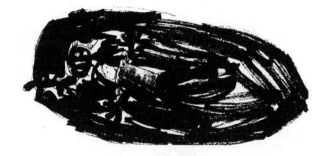

I lost my cat Bear bear, I was really sad And I buried her. I mist her alot and when I start crying I go in my room and I get her collar and I hold it in my hand or I put it under my pillow and it calms me down.

Figure 9.12 This child developed a wonderful coping skill for working through a loss. A child's keeping the pet's collar, holding it, and sleeping with it under the pillow are excellent ways to comfort a child. The collar is a link to the life shared with the pet–a tangible keepsake.

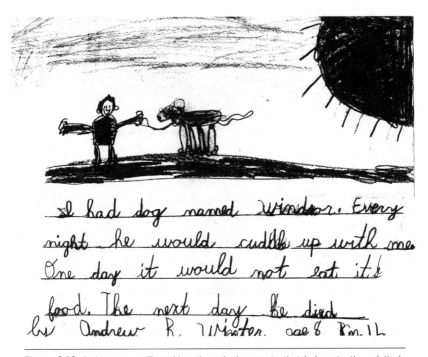

Figure 9.13 Andrew was still working through the events that led up to the relatively sudden loss of his dog Windsor.

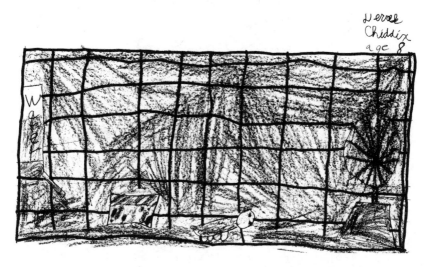

One time I went to see my hamster and I tapped on his cage and I thought that he was sleeping. A couple of days later I went to see my dad and he said "Hamster was dedd" and I was very sad.

Figure 9.14

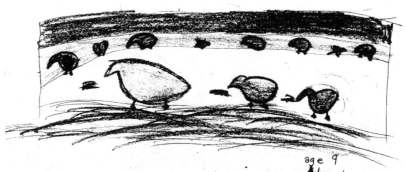

When I was little I had chicks. I always kept
them warm. I named them Shey, Cutie, & Tricky. I played
with every chick. With Cutie I hugged him. With Shey was really
fun to play with, Tricky was tricky because she always
ran away from me when I hugged her.

But one day all of them died. I cried a llot
When my 3 chicks died. I remember my
three chicks, my hugging their blanket that they used,
I miss Shey, Cutie, Tricky.

age 9
Alondra Mendez

Figure 9.15

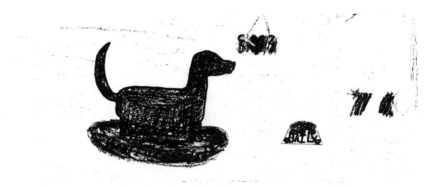

When my dog Bailey died I felt
very sad because she was a very
loyal and very important part of our
family. I liked her eyes and her beautiful
hair.

                                        Janae Hallinan age 9

Figure 9.16

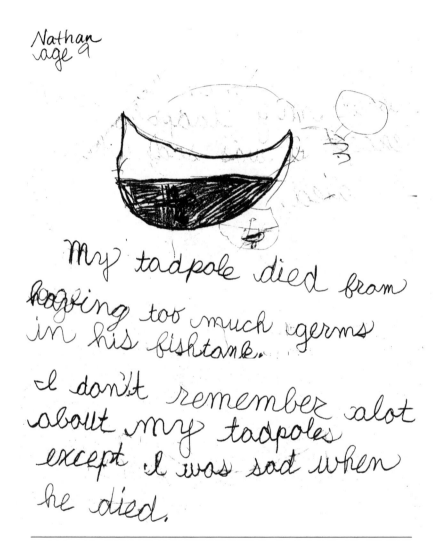

Nathan
age 9

My tadpole died from
hagsing too much germs
in his fishtank.

I don't remember alot
about my tadpoles
except I was sad when
he died.

Figure 9.17 The bond Nathan shared with his tadpole is a testament that the loss of even the smallest, seemingly insignificant creatures can be experienced as significant by the child who loves and cares for them.

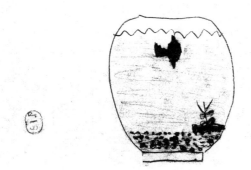

I had a fish named Sharky
I felt Sad when he died. I liked his
strips and I liked him

Figure 9.18 Dustin Hallinan, age 7.

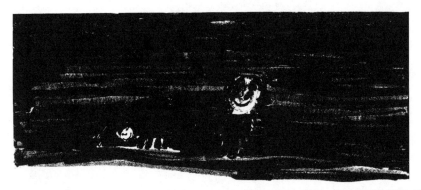

One time my cat died. I felt very sad.
It was very sweet. At night it jumped up on you
bed and curled up at the end it. My cat was a boy
and its name was Simon. It was about 14 years old. When I
think about Simon I feel very sad. There is othing that helps
me. What helps me is I think about the world and think that I have more
things than I don't have. That was very sad for me. Demi Matthews Age 9

Figure 9.19

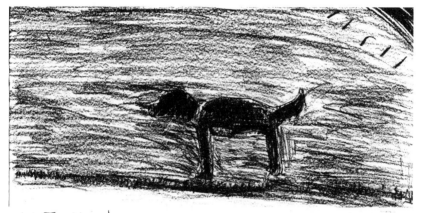

I had a dog named Sammy. She died on my birthday. When she died I was so sad. I remember her by looking at a picture of her.
SARAH Otten 9

Figure 9.20 Often when a pet's death occurs on or near an important date, a child can experience mixed emotions about a joyful occasion, such as a birthday, and sadness at the loss of the pet for years to come. Helping the child to remember the date as a celebration of life—a birthday and the life shared with the pet—can assist the child in continuing to work through the loss by acknowledging the loss in a positive way on a happy occasion.

Bobo

by Irene Van Riper, seventh grade

Dear, dear Mr. Bobo
The king of cats
He thought he was human
Even when he napped
Sprawled out on the lawn,
Yawned, got comfy
Then went to sleep
With one eye open
He expected his meals
Promptly at eight—
And if we late—
Watch out,
He'd become a lion.
Would meow and hiss
If you picked him up –
A very touchy cat, I must admit.
He knew his brands,
Only the finest food would suffice.
No Albertsons, Safeway or Costco for him
We had to go 50 miles for him!
Yes, San Francisco, I believe was his liking,
But with all those hardships
Yes, I must admit
Bobo was pretty fine in the end.
Bobo the great, Bobo the brave,
Bobo the cute, Bobo is Bobo!
But Bobo is no longer with us (*sniff*)
As sad as it is, we have to move on
For Bobo will always be with us in spirit.

My Best Friend

by Katie Conley, seventh grade

Have you ever had a pet that was your best friend? A golden retriever/black lab was the greatest and truest friend anyone could ever find. He became such a big part of my life that when he had to go, a part of me was lost forever.

He never lost his puppy fur, so if one touched his long black silky fur one would believe he was an over-grown puppy. Besides his white whiskers, his years were hidden from view with his never-ending smile. Snickers' love was so great that you could feel the warmth of it by just entering the same room he was in. His love never weakened even in his last few breaths.

"Paper may be more patient than man" but paper is not more patient than my best friend Snickers. He always pleased anyone near him with his simple ways. He even acted like he was married to me by following the promise "through sickness and health, til death do us part." He never left my side after I was brought home from the hospital. Even as I was leaving his head was gently lying on my lap. His slow steady breathing seemed to be trying to comfort me by saying, "I may be leaving physically but I will never leave your side spiritually.:

Sometimes I can feel my hands running through his fluffy fur. I can still feel the warmth of his love but instead of being in the air, it is located inside of me. I can't help but notice the small similarities that Snickers and other dogs possess. The only things that I have not seen in other dogs are his love and his patience.

10

RESOURCES FOR HELPING CHILDREN AND THEIR FAMILIES THROUGH PET LOSS

Education is not the filling of a pail but the lighting of a fire.
—William Butler Yeats

We read to know that we are not alone. Through education we gain knowledge. Knowing where and whom to go to during a time of loss can provide us with the tools to best help our clients and our children. Reaching out to others in times of distress is not only wise, it is healthy and provides us with the tools we need to work through heartfelt emotions and to learn to trust to love again. There are many resources available to caregivers. Provided in this chapter is a reading list for therapists, parents, teachers, and anyone who works with and cares for children of books for children, Web sites, pet loss support hotlines, universities, and other grief resources on a national and international level.

Resources

American Psychological Association
http://www.apa.org

Pet Loss Support Hotlines and Grief Counselor Referral Web Sites

College of Veterinary Medicine, University of Illinois at
Urbana–Champaign
C.A.R.E. Pet Loss Helpline
1-877-394-2273
griefhelp@cvm.uiuc.edu

Delta Society
580 Naches Avenue SW, Suite 101
Renton, WA 98055-2297
425-226-7357
info@deltasociety.org
www.deltasociety.org

The Delta Society contains a list of pet loss and bereavement
resources.

Center for Companion Animal Behavior
School of Veterinary Medicine
University of California Davis
http://www.vetmed.ucdavis.edu/ccab/petloss.html

The Center for Companion Animal Behavior lists memori-
als, hotlines, and organizational and Web resources for companion animal loss.

International Association of Pet Cemeteries
Pet Loss Support Hotline
518-594-3000

Washington State University
College of Veterinary Medicine
Pullman, VA
509-335-5704

Trained Washington State University veterinary student vol-
unteers staff the phones as compassionate listeners from 6:30
P.M. to 9:00 P.M. (Pacific time) Monday through Thursday
and 1:00 P.M. to 3:00 P.M. on Saturdays.

P.A.T.S. (Pet Loss Support Line)
Pacific Animal Therapy Society
9412 Lauries' Lane
Sidney, B.C., V8L 4L2, Canada
250-389-8047

The Pet Loss Support Hotline
Iowa State University
2116 College of Veterinary Medicine
Ames, IA 50011
888-478-7574

Pet Loss Support Hotline
University of Florida
College of Veterinary Medicine
Gainsville, FL
352-392-4700, ext. 4080

Pet Loss Support Hotline
Tufts University
Boston, MA
508-839-7966
www.tufts.edu/vet/petloss

Pet Loss Support Hotline
Companion Animal Hospital
Box 35
College of Veterinary Medicine
Cornell University
Ithaca, NY 14853-6401
607-253-3932
www.vet.cornell.edu/public/petloss

The Ohio State University Pet Loss Hotline
614-292-1823

Pet Loss Support Hotline
Virginia–Maryland Regional College of Veterinary Medicine
540-231-8038

Pet Grief Support Service
Companion Animal Association of Arizona Inc.
P.O. Box 5006
Scottsdale, AZ
602-995-5885

Pet Loss Support Program
Michigan State University
College of Veterinary Medicine
Clinical Center C-100
East Lansing, MI 48824
517-353-5064

The Chicago Veterinary Medical Association Pet Loss Support
Helpline
630-325-1600

Argus Institute for Families and Veterinary Medicine
College of Veterinary Medicine and Biomedical Sciences
Colorado State University
970-297-4143

Hawaiian Human Society
http://www.hawaiianhumane.org

University of Minnesota School of Veterinary Medicine Pet
Loss Support Hotline
612-625-3770

The Association for Pet Loss Bereavement (APLB)
P.O. Box 106
Brooklyn, NY 11230

718-382-0690
http://www.aplb.org

Maintains a comprehensive directory of therapists who have special training or interest in pet loss

The University of Pennsylvania
School of Veterinary Medicine
Philadelphia, PA
212-898-4529

The Rainbow Passage Pet Loss Support and Bereavement Center
Grafton, WI
414-376-0340

The Australian Center for Companion Animals in Society
(02) 9746 1911

Pet Bereavement Support Service (England)
0800-096-6606

Super Dog Pet Loss Support and Grief Counseling
http://www.superdog.com/petloss/counsel.htm

Lists grief counselors throughout the United States

The Iams Pet Loss Support Center and Hotline
888-332-7738

American Veterinary Medical Association
Pet Loss Resources
http://www.avma.org/care4pets/avmaloss.htm

For support groups and hotlines not listed in your area, contact your local or state veterinary medical association.

EMDR Resources

David Grand, Ph.D.
2415 Jerusalem Avenue
Suite 105
Bellmore, NY 11710
516-785-0460
Dgrand1952@aol.com
http://www.biolateral.com/bio.htm

Francine Shapiro, Ph.D.
http://www.emdr.com/shapiro.htm

EMDR: Eye Movement Desensitization and Reprocessing: Basic Principles, Protocols and Procedures (New York: Guilford, 2001); *EMDR: The Breakthrough Therapy for Overcoming Anxiety, Stress and Trauma* (New York: Basic Books, 1997); and *EMDR as an Integrative Psychotherapy Approach: Experts of Diverse Orientations Explore the Paradigm Prism* (Washington, DC: American Psychological Association Books, 2002).

EMDR: A Closer Look. Guilford Press Video, New York, 1998. http://www.guilford.com

Books for Adults

Antinori, Deborah. *Journey Through Pet Loss*. Yoko Spirit Publishers. www.petlossaudio.com.

Axline, Virginia M. *Play Therapy*. New York: Ballantine Books, 1947.

Butler, C. *The Human-Animal Bond and Grief.*

Carmack, Betty J. *Grieving the Death of a Pet*. Minneapolis, MN: Ausberg Fortress, 2003.

Goldman, Linda. *Breaking the Silence*. New York: Brunner-Routledge, 2001.

Goldman, Linda. *Life and Loss: A Guide to Help Grieving Children*. New York: Taylor and Francis, 2000.

Kay, William J. *Pet Loss and Human Bereavement.* Ames: Iowa State University Press, 1984.

Levy, T. *Attachment, Trauma, and Healing: Understanding and Treating Attachment Disorder in Children and Families.* Washington, DC: CWLA Press, 1998.

McElroy, Susan Chernak. *Animals as Teachers and Healers.* New York: Ballantine Books, 1996.

Nieberg, H. A., & A. Fisher. *Pet Loss: A Thoughtful Guide for Adults and Children.* New York: Harper & Row, 1982.

Polland, Barbara Kay. *Feelings: Inside You and Outloud Too.* Berkeley, CA: Ten Speed Press, 1997.

Reynolds, Rebecca A. *Bring Me the Ocean: Nature as Teacher, Messenger, and Intermediary.* Acton, MA: VanderWyk & Burnham, 1995.

Ross, Cheri Barton, and Jane Baron-Sorensen. *Pet Loss and Human Emotion: Guiding Clients Through Grief.* Philadelphia, PA: Accelerated Development, 1998.

Tousley, M. *Children and Pet Loss: A Guide for Helping.* Phoenix: Companion Animal Association Arizona, Our Pals Publishing Company, 1996.

Traisman, Enid Samuel. *My Personal Pet Remembrance Journal.* Wenatchee, WA: Dove Lewis Emergency Animal, Direct Book Services, 1996.

Wolfelt, Alan. *Children and Grief.* Philadelphia, PA: Accelerated Development, 1983.

Books for Children

Blain, M. *Jasper's Day.* Toronto, ON Canada: Kids Can Press, 2002.

Rogers, Fred. *When a Pet Dies.* New York: G. P. Putnam, 1988.

Rylant, C. *Dog Heaven.* New York: Blue Sky PRess, Scholastic, Inc., 1995.

Rylant, C. *Cat Heaven.* New York: Blue Sky PRess, Scholastic, Inc., 1997.

Voirst, J. *The Tenth Good Thing About Barney.* New York: Aladdin Paperbacks, Simon & Schuster, 1971.

NOTES

Chapter 1

1. Terry M. Levy and Michael Orlans, *Attachment, Trauma and Healing: Understanding and Treating Attachment Disorder in Children and Families* (Washington, DC: Child Welfare League of America, 1998).
2. Alan Wolfelt, *Helping Children Cope With Grief* (Philadelphia, PA: Accelerated Development, 1988), 52–53.
3. Ibid., 54.
4. Sandi Martin, "Goodbye Friend: Meeting the Needs of Yourself and Others Impacted by the Loss of Your Therapy Animal," Delta Society Conference Proceedings, May 16, 2003, Seattle, WA.
5. Valentine Davies, *Miracle on 34th Street* (New York: Harcourt, 1947), 116.
6. Elisabeth Kübler-Ross, *On Death and Dying* (New York: COllier, 1969).
7. See Cheri Barton Ross and Jane Baron-Sorensen, *Pet Loss and Human Emotion: Guiding Clients Through Grief* (Philadelphia, PA: Accelerated Development, 1998), 16.
8. *In America,* written and directed by Jim Sheridan (2003).
9. Ross and Baron-Sorensen, *Pet Loss and Human Emotion,* 73–74.
10. Linda Goldman, *Breaking the Silence* (New York: Brunner-Routledge, 2001).

Chapter 2

1. Carl R. Rogers, *Client Centered Therapy: It's Current Practice, Implications, and Theory* (Trans-Atlantic Publications, 1995, Reprint Edition), 52.
2. Ibid., 49.
3. Terry M. Levy and Michael Orlans, *Attachment, Trauma and Healing: Understanding and Treating Attachment Disorder in Children and Families* (Washington, DC: Child Welfare League of America, 1998), 226.
4. Cheri Barton Ross and Jane Baron-Sorensen, *Pet Loss and Human Emotion: Guiding Clients Through Grief* (Philadelphia, PA: Accelerated Development, 1998).
5. Ibid., 69-70.

6. M. Tousley, *Children and Pet Loss: A Guide for Helping* (Phoenix: Companion Animal Association Arizona, Our Pals Publishing Company, 1996), 15.
7. *Houseboat.* Directed by Melville Shaverlson. Paramount Pictures, 1958.

Chapter 3

1. Marjorie Blain Parker, *Jasper's Day* (Tonawanda, NY: Kids Can Press, 2002).
2. Cheri Barton Ross and Jane Baron-Sorensen, *Pet Loss and Human Emotion: Guiding Clients Through Grief* (Philadelphia, PA: Accelerated Development, 1998).
3. Enid Samuel Traisman, *My Personal Pet Remembrance Journal* (Wenatchee, WA: Dove Lewis Emergency Animal, Direct Book Services, 1996).
4. Judith Voirst, *The Tenth Good Thing About Barney* (New York: Aladdin Paperbacks, Simon & Schuster, 1971).
5. See Ross and Baron-Sorensen, *Pet Loss and Human Emotion,* 75-76.

Chapter 4

1. Cheri Barton Ross and Jane Baron-Sorensen, *Pet Loss and Human Emotion: Guiding Clients Through Grief* (Philadelphia, PA: Accelerated Development, 1998).
2. Susan Chernak McElory, *Animals as Teachers and Healers* (New York: Ballantine Books, 1996).
3. Ibid., 182.

Chapter 5

1. H. A. Neiburg and A. Fisher, *Pet Loss: A Thoughtful Guide for Adults and Children* (New York: Harper & Row, 1982), 80.
2. Cheri Barton Ross and Jane Baron-Sorensen, *Pet Loss and Human Emotion: Guiding Clients Through Grief* (Philadelphia, PA: Accelerated Development, 1998), 103.
3. L. Lagoni, C. Butler, and S. Hetts, *The Human-Animal Bond and Grief* (Philadelphia: W. B. Saunders, 1994).

Chapter 8

1. Virginia M. Axline, *Play Therapy,* rev. ed. (New York: Ballantine Books, 1969), 182–183.
2. Ibid., 58.
3. Mark A. Nemiroff, Jane Annunziata, and Margaret Scott, *A Child's First Book About Play Therapy* (American Psychological Association, Nov. 1, 1990) 71.
4. Ibid., 38.
5. Nemiroff and Annunziata (1990), 26.
6. Barbara Kay Polland, *Feelings: Inside You and Outloud Too* (Berkeley, CA: Ten Speed Press, 1997).

7. Jane Annunziata, *Play Therapy With a Six Year Old,* APA Online Videos.
8. Kathy McBeth. <info@instituteforchildren.com>
9. Cheri Barton Ross and Jane Baron-Sorensen, *Pet Loss and Human Emotion: Guiding Clients Through Grief* (Philadelphia, PA: Accelerated Development, 1998), 145-46.
10. Ricky Greenwald, "Applying Eye Movement Desensitization and Reprocessing (EMDR) to the Treatment of Traumatized Children: Five Case Studies." <http://www.childtrauma.com>
11. Jon G. Allen, Michael W. Keller, and David A. Console, *EMDR: A Closer Look,* Video manual (New York, London: Guilford, 1999).
12. Ricky Greenwald, *Anxiety Disorders Practice Journal* 1 (1994): 83-97.
13. Ibid.
14. Ricky Greenwald, *EMDR: A New Treatment for Traumatic Memories* (Childhood Trauma Institute). <http://www.childtrauma.com> Updated October 13, 1999.

INDEX